the
midlife
method

Sam Rice is a freelance food and health writer and the author of *The Midlife Kitchen*, a *Sunday Times* bestseller she wrote with fellow food writer and journalist Mimi Spencer. Sam's journey into healthy living began in 2012 when her youngest brother died suddenly from complications arising from Type 1 diabetes. This was a catalyst for change: in the process of overhauling her own lifestyle, Sam began to research and write about midlife weight management and health. *The Midlife Method* is the result.

Sam is also a qualified oenologist and wine writer and holds a Wine & Spirit Education Trust diploma. After moving to Bali with her family in 2013, she was the wine columnist for *Inspired Bali* magazine. These days, Sam lives in Singapore with her husband and two teenage children. She is a regular contributor to a number of print and online publications and has a monthly column in *Top Santé* magazine. She has recently been accepted into the Guild of Food Writers.

The nutritional consultant for *The Midlife Method*, Sarah Schenker, is one of the UK's leading dietitians. She is further qualified as an accredited sports dietitian and registered public health nutritionist. Sarah has a wealth of experience as a health writer and broadcaster, and regularly contributes to titles as diverse as the *Daily Mail*, *The Times*, *Men's Health*, *Cosmopolitan*, *Glamour* and *Top Santé*. She has also appeared on TV, including *This Morning*, *Live with Gabby*, *Watchdog*, *Sky News* and across national and local BBC radio. Sarah worked with Sam as the nutritional advisor on *The Midlife Kitchen*. She is also a member of the Association for Nutrition, the Nutrition Society and the Guild of Health Writers, and has served on professional and government committees.

the
midlife
method

How to lose weight and feel great after 40

SAM RICE

with registered dietitian
Sarah Schenker

The author has a Certificate in Nutrition certified by the Association for Nutrition in the UK and for this book she worked with Sarah Schenker, a UK registered dietitian, to ensure that the plan is safe, evidence-based, and in line with current healthy eating guidelines. However, the weight loss programme and meal plans may not be suitable for everyone to follow, especially those with an underlying medical condition or food-related disorder. The information contained in this book is not intended to be a substitute for medical advice or medical treatment.

You are advised to consult a doctor on any matters relating to your health, and in particular on any matters that may require diagnosis or medical attention. Do not stop or change any prescription medications without the guidance and advice of your doctor. Any use of the information in this book is made on the reader's good judgement after consulting with their doctor, and is the reader's sole responsibility.

First published in 2020 by Headline Home
an imprint of Headline Publishing Group

3

ISBN 978 1 4722 7893 7
eISBN 978 1 4722 7894 4

Publishing Director: Lindsey Evans
Senior Editor: Kate Miles
Copy editors: Jane Hammett and Tara O'Sullivan
Proofreaders: Sally Sargeant and Margaret Gilbey
Indexer: Caroline Wilding

Designed and typeset by EM&EN
Printed and bound in Great Britain by Clays Ltd, Elcograf S.p.A.

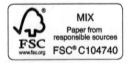

MIX
Paper from
responsible sources
FSC® C104740

HEADLINE PUBLISHING GROUP
An Hachette UK Company
Carmelite House
50 Victoria Embankment
London EC4Y 0DZ

www.headline.co.uk
www.hachette.co.uk

For Ben

Contents

Foreword

When we reach midlife, a curious alchemy of time and gravity contrives to slow us all down a bit. Joints sometimes ache. A layer of comfort cushioning takes up unwelcome residence where a summer midriff used to be. We start to be secretly fascinated by our changing eyelids and jowls, by the backs of our hands and the shape of our knees – things we barely noticed a few years ago.

Dealing well with ageing requires a strategy to sustain ourselves, both physically and mentally, as the years roll by. Most of us will need a gentle rethink of our approach to diet, sleep, stress management and exercise, guided by a fresh understanding of what's happening to our metabolism, our hormones and our digestion. Some of us will benefit from advice about how to mitigate against conditions typically associated with ageing, such as osteoporosis, diabetes and cognitive decline. At 40 and beyond, we all need a roadmap to get us from A to B – that hazardous path through the middle years – in the best possible shape.

When Sam and I worked so happily together on *The Midlife Kitchen*, we always held as a central intent the need to *embrace* midlife: to be wholeheartedly pro-ageing, not anti-ageing. Sam's new book sets out a plan to facilitate that embrace. Her promise is that we can all discover health, happiness and – yes – weight loss in midlife by developing a positive relationship with food.

Through her own experience as someone who, like many of us, had always wanted to be 'that bit slimmer', Sam has devised a practical and enjoyable weight-loss protocol that deftly condenses the latest research and thinking around fundamentals such as eating with awareness, implementing portion control and fostering healthy habits around food. There's plenty of practical guidance here, together with simple, delicious and satisfying recipes and meal plans to fit seamlessly into a busy life.

The Midlife Method is a fantastic philosophy for living well. It's a method for people who enjoy food but who want to put it gently in its place. It's for anyone looking for a clearly signed path to healthy eating and a happy weight in midlife and beyond. Sam's set of simple messages can be imported into any life – not just for a month, not just for a year, but forever. I can't think of a better reason to dig in.

Mimi Spencer, co-author of *The Fast Diet* and *The Midlife Kitchen*

Welcome to the Midlife Method

As a food and health writer and recipe creator, I've long understood that the way to successful weight management is through good, nutritious food – but sometimes simply eating well isn't enough to lose weight. Once we hit midlife, things change: our hormones become depleted and erratic and our metabolism begins to slow. Muscle mass also starts to decrease, and our gut becomes less efficient at extracting what we need from our food. In short, we need more nutrition from fewer calories. Midlife weight loss is no cakewalk.

My first book *The Midlife Kitchen*, written with my good friend Mimi Spencer, who also kindly contributed the foreword for this book, was one of the first food books to recognise that in our middle years we need a different approach to nutrition. Mimi and I had noticed, as we progressed through our forties, that we no longer craved the carb-heavy foods that had dominated our dinner plates through our twenties and thirties. Food was no longer simply a way of fuelling ourselves through the day, but of responding to our changing nutritional requirements; our bodies were telling us we needed to eat differently. We wrote *The Midlife Kitchen* to address that need – a cookbook full of delicious food that would satisfy our changing midlife palates.

And I know we're not alone. I speak to fellow midlifers every day who have also noticed a shift in appetite: they are now more drawn to an interesting salad than a slice of pizza. This is good news because a healthy diet is the foundation of a longer, more active life – and the key to reducing our risk of age-related diseases.

The problem comes when, despite our best efforts, we find weight accumulating around our middles. A 'WTF?' moment, one might say.

While *The Midlife Kitchen* was concerned with eating well to support health in midlife, *The Midlife Method* takes the next step. It addresses the issue of midlife weight loss. Although eating healthily is of paramount importance, we need to keep an eye on the scales if we want to maximise our chances of good health in later years. It's well known that being overweight is one of the main risk factors for the 'big five' chronic diseases: cardiovascular disease, Type 2 diabetes, chronic respiratory disease, cancer and stroke. In midlife, this is no longer something we can afford to ignore.

So, if you are a fellow midlifer and you've found that weight is creeping on, or perhaps you feel that you're eating well but your waistline is not responding, this book is for you.

Midlife weight loss is indeed a challenge, but it is possible, and the way to do it can be found in these pages.

My story

In August 2012 my youngest brother Ben died, aged 27. He had Type 1 diabetes, and many health complications as a result. At the time I was a 42-year-old mother of two young children and my own health was not a priority. With Ben's death, that changed. My brother had been robbed of his once healthy body; I owed it to him to take better care of mine.

I wasn't vastly overweight – probably a stone more than I wanted to be – but let's just say my jeans were very snug. I'd tried loads of diets in the past, even a stint on those depressing meal replacement shakes, and I *had* lost weight . . . but inevitably, once the diet was over, the pounds crept back on.

I was also getting more and more confused about what I should be eating. One minute I read that this food was good for me, the next it was bad. Everything I ate seemed wrong: it had too much fat, or salt, or it was full of chemicals, which made me feel guilty for eating it. Food had somehow become the enemy.

And I was also getting older. I had 'hit the middle' and my body wasn't playing ball. After a week of trying to 'be good', the scales would barely respond. I needed a plan to help me make the right food choices – but without having to devote masses of mental energy to everything I ate. There was no workable framework out there for my life as a busy midlife mother.

That was eight years ago. It has been a gradual process of re-education, research, nutritional study and time spent in the kitchen to get to where I am today. It has ignited in me a passion for healthy eating that I could never have predicted, and has led to a new career as a food and health writer. I did eventually lose that stone and, once I had lost it, my new understanding of how and what to eat helped me to keep it off. I had made friends with food again.

Losing weight at any stage of life requires focus, determination and patience, and *The Midlife Method* is no different. There is no magic potion we can take that will do the work for us but, in the absence of an underlying medical condition, if you commit to this programme for 28 days you will lose weight and, more importantly, have the knowledge to manage your weight in the future.

The simple, delicious recipes I have created for the meal plans in this book are nutritionally balanced to support optimum health in midlife. I have tried to make them as family-friendly as possible so that you can still all eat together, especially at dinner time.

You owe it to yourself – and your loved ones – to look after your body, lose that weight, and live your best midlife. If I can do it, so can you. Here's how.

Introduction

What is your motivation?

This is probably the most important question to ask yourself before embarking on any weight-loss programme. So, let's think about it for a moment.

I'm assuming, because you have bought this book, you are most likely a Generation X-er like me, born between the early 1960s and the late 1970s. You're old enough to remember the Cabbage Soup Diet and Jane Fonda in her snazzy leotards, but young enough to still bother dyeing your roots.

Little did we know back then, as we bopped around our bedrooms to Duran Duran, watching in horror as the space shuttle *Challenger* blew up (and in delight as the Berlin Wall came down), that we were destined to become the diet industry's guinea pigs. Throughout the 1990s and 2000s we pushed hard on the glass ceiling and tried to 'have it all', but at the same time we were unknowingly being enslaved by the tyranny of being thin. (Men reading this book, you are lucky enough to belong to the last generation of males who weren't under any social pressure to look good!)

There was a constant background fear that our bodies weren't good enough, that we'd be so much happier/cooler/more attractive (delete as appropriate) if we could *just be thinner*. Supermodels were held up as ideals for us to emulate. I remember marvelling at Cindy Crawford's slim, perfectly oiled thighs as I puffed along to her workout video – and she was the 'fat' supermodel! Then along came Kate Moss with her 'heroin chic' look, announcing to a generation of women that 'nothing tastes as good as skinny feels'. We had a lot on our plates – or so we were told.

Old habits die hard, and it would be disingenuous of me to say that vanity plays no part in my wanting to keep my weight under control as I head into my fifties. But one of the things I have noticed about getting older – and most of my midlife mates concur – is that we accept that our bodies are changing. To a certain degree, that's OK; it's simply nature taking its course. The perfection we used to covet is no longer within our grasp; our focus has subtly shifted from better booties to better microbiomes. Even Jane Fonda agrees: 'We're not meant to be perfect. It took me a long time to learn that'.[1]

So, back to the motivation question. Yes, many midlifers still want to be thinner but, increasingly, losing weight for us is about prolonging our health span: that is, the number of fit, active and healthy years we have ahead of us. This sentiment was neatly expressed by my mother who, when reading an early version of this book, commented as follows:

> As an older person, it seems that the younger me did not really believe that the older me would ever arrive, and I didn't care about her! All those 'lifestyle' diseases – heart problems, stroke, Type 2 diabetes – can be delayed, or even avoided, by eating well and keeping your weight under control. Also, you will be more mobile and more able to enjoy the activities you love for longer.

These are compelling reasons for managing our weight as we age, but surely everything there is to say about weight loss has already been said, right? You either have to cut out certain things (fat, carbs, grains, gluten, dairy . . .) or eat within specific times (5:2 or 16:8 . . .) or eat a plant-based diet, or . . . actually, what is it we should be doing?

You may have noticed that the title of this book is not *The Midlife Diet* but *The Midlife Method* – and therein lies the clue. Midlife weight loss has to be holistic. Simply eating less will lead to weight loss in the short term but it will not be sustainable over the long term – and if it's not sustainable, then what's the point?

Also, we do ourselves no good by simply cutting things out of our diet with no understanding of the nutrition our bodies require to stay healthy. Let's revisit our motivation for a second: it's not just about dropping a dress size any more. Sure, we want to lose weight, but we also want to feel great.

So where do we start? Let's look at the weight-loss question first. Calorie deficit – the technical term for consuming less energy than you expend – is the only proven way to lose weight. All weight-loss programmes, no matter how they are packaged, have this at their core. So does the Midlife Method – because, to repeat, *it is the only proven way to lose weight*. But if we want to lose weight healthily, we need to ensure that, at the same time as losing weight, we're providing our bodies with the nutrition they need to function well. For any weight loss to be sustainable, it must be underpinned by healthy habits: regular exercise, good sleep, stress management, and low to moderate alcohol intake (if you drink).

This book will show you how to do this. The Midlife Method is a 28-day plan based on the concept of Light Days, where we calorie restrict, and Regular Days, where we eat normally but learn to make better food choices to support weight management in the future. Unlike many diets, nothing is cut out altogether; all food groups are welcome at the Midlife Method's table and there are no restrictions around when to eat. Not a breakfast fan? Fine – eat later. Prefer to eat a big lunch and a smaller dinner? No problem. If family dinners are important to you, make them your main meal of the day.

When the four weeks are over, you'll have changed not just how much and what you eat (and all the recipes are delicious, I promise), but also how you approach exercise, sleep, stress and alcohol. Our bodies change in midlife and so must we. Using the Midlife Method, we can.

Are you ready for change?

Losing weight involves behavioural change. Studies have shown that, for change to be successful, the most important factor is motivation. People are motivated to change their behaviour when they understand the problems it causes, they are concerned about its effects, and they feel positive and confident that they can change. The following elements are required:

Knowledge of the potential problems caused by their behaviour: We will cover this in the next section, Why is midlife weight loss so important?

Concern about the effects on themselves and others: You are pre-qualified by virtue of the fact you have bought this book!

Being confident in their ability to implement the required changes: I sincerely hope that this book will empower you to make the lifestyle changes you need to achieve your goal.

It is crucial, therefore, that before starting the Midlife Method, you are fully committed to change. For the next four weeks you will need to make what you eat and your well-being your top priority. You will need to plan meals, find time to exercise, and address any other lifestyle issues you may have, such as sleep, stress or alcohol intake. All are necessary to kick-start the weight-loss process – and for long-term success.

So, for the next few weeks put yourself first. You will need time, energy and a positive mindset to make the lifestyle changes necessary to lose those unwanted pounds – and, more importantly, to keep them off.

Why is midlife weight loss so important?

Weight management, at any time of life, is important for your overall health, but studies show that obesity from our middle years onwards is one of the main risk factors for a range of chronic diseases. A UK observational study[2] based on the NHS records of 2.8 million people found that those who were severely obese in middle age (with a body mass index, or BMI, over 35) were 50% more likely to die early than those of a healthy weight. Even those with a lower BMI (30–35) had twice the risk of having high blood pressure and nearly twice the risk of heart failure than those with a normal BMI. This is just the latest of a number of studies linking obesity to poor long-term health outcomes.

A recent review conducted by the Mayo Clinic,[3] an academic medical research organisation based in the USA, indicated that being overweight is of particular concern to menopausal women. According to the study, weight gain – accompanied by an increased tendency towards central fat distribution – can result in adverse metabolic consequences, including problems regulating sugar and fat levels in the blood, high blood pressure and cardiovascular disease. The report states: 'Given that cardiovascular disease is the leading cause of death in postmenopausal women, the importance of weight management in midlife cannot be overemphasised' (p. 1552).

In addition, for both men and women, obesity is one of the main contributing factors to developing dementia and Alzheimer's disease in later life.[4]

More recently, obesity has been in the spotlight because of the Covid-19 pandemic. At the time of writing, studies show a strong correlation between obesity and an increased risk of dying from Covid-19. Hospitalised coronavirus patients classified as obese (with a BMI of more than 30) have a 33% greater risk of dying than those who are not.[5]

Unfortunately, weight gain is all too common among midlifers: menopausal women gain on average about 1.5 pounds (0.7kg) per year during their forties and fifties, and there seems to be a similar pattern for men. The most recent UK government figures[6] suggested that 70% of people in the UK aged over 45 are overweight or obese.

Add to this the more recent spike in weight gain as a result of coronavirus lockdowns around the world – the 'quarantine 15', as it has become known, referring to an average 15lb weight increase – and it doesn't take a genius to figure out that obesity is a ticking time bomb for public health.

Apart from the risks to our future health, there are other downsides to being overweight, not least the negative impact it has on our self-esteem. I don't wish to discuss the rights or wrongs of society's 'fattitude' – that's the subject of a book in itself. Suffice to say, in our Western society, and increasingly in other cultures, there is a positive moral value attached to thinness. This is summarised very well by Dr Meg Arroll and Louise Atkinson in their excellent book *The Shrinkology Solution*:

> Food science, advertising and marketing have become a highly specialised force which cleverly tempts us to buy and consume food we might not really want or need. We'd be mad to underestimate its power. This effect is magnified by the inexorable rise of social media. Together these additional pressures subtly persuade us that what we eat and our body shape and size define us. (Chapter 2)[7]

Apart from societal pressure to be thinner, the practical limitations of being overweight can also affect our quality of life. The heavier we are, the less mobile we become, and the less inclined we are to exercise – it's a vicious cycle of weight gain, reduced mobility, less exercise, more weight gain, further reduced mobility, even less exercise, and so it goes on. Add to this other age-related issues such as bone and joint pain, poor sleep or the stress of juggling work, parenting teens and looking after elderly relatives, and it really is the perfect health storm.

So far, so depressing. Sorry, but here's the good news – you don't have to be a statistic. The study of longevity genes is a developing science, but it is estimated that only about 25% of the variation in human lifespan is determined by genetics.[8] That means the rest, a whopping 75%, is down to environmental factors.

And that's where the Midlife Method comes in. Based on research into the specific challenges we face when it comes to weight management in midlife, the Midlife Method is a holistic programme that helps us to change the way we eat, and also helps us to support weight loss with other lifestyle interventions. Exercise, sleep, stress and alcohol all pay a crucial part in the midlife weight-loss conundrum, so we need to address any issues we have in these areas if we wish to lose weight healthily and sustainably.

Making changes now can help us to alter the course of our future. So, let's do ourselves – and the NHS – a favour: there has never been a better time in our lives to lose weight and feel great.

What is a healthy weight?

We need to make a distinction here between what is considered a 'healthy weight' in a medical sense, and the weight we would actually like to be. If you look at the NHS healthy weight chart (Figure 1), you'll see that, based on your height, there is quite a wide range of values that is considered a 'healthy weight'. Assessing weight in terms of height is rather a crude method, but it is a useful tool to see if we are in the right ballpark, and serves as a starting point for thinking about our target weight.

What is BMI?

Body mass index (BMI) is a mathematical formula that divides a person's weight by the square of their height. The main limitation of this measure is that you end up with a single value that *is* your BMI. Whether you are underweight, overweight or obese is decided by that figure. BMI is not reliable when applied to, say, elderly adults who have generally lost some muscle and bone mass. An elderly person's BMI could be within a normal range, while they might actually be carrying too much body fat.

The healthy weight chart in Figure 1 also compares height and weight. Because it provides a generous healthy weight range, we can take other factors (such as age, genetics and weight history) into account when deciding what constitutes a healthy, achievable target weight for an individual.

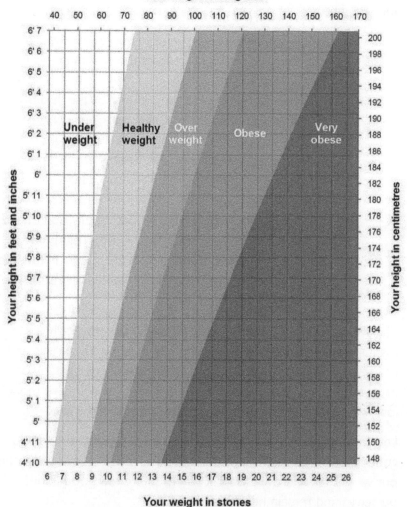

Figure 1. The NHS healthy weight chart.

From https://www.nhs.uk/live-well/healthy-weight/height-weight-chart/

To set a realistic and sustainable target weight, ask yourself:

- What is the lightest I have ever been in my adult life?
- What is the heaviest I have ever been in my adult life (not including pregnancies)?

Referring to the weight chart, look up the healthy weight range for your height, then:

- If, at your very lightest, you were in the 'overweight' to 'very obese' part of the chart, take the maximum healthy weight for your height.
- If you have hovered around the top end of the 'healthy weight' range and possibly a bit over, set your sights somewhere just over midway in the 'healthy weight' range.
- If you have wandered all over the 'healthy weight' range, aim for a weight around the middle of the range.
- If, at your heaviest, you were around the middle or lower part of the 'healthy weight' range, you actually don't need to lose weight, but you can still follow this programme if you just want to lose a pound or two, or simply follow the Regular Days section of the Midlife Method to ensure you're eating a healthy, balanced diet.

The weight at which each of us feels good, both physically and mentally, is a very personal thing, but we need to be realistic and not set a goal that is unsustainable. If you are overweight, a good initial target is to lose 5% of your body weight. If you have more to lose, you can always set a new goal further down the line.

Let's face it: weight loss in midlife is no longer just about looking good in a swimsuit (although that would be nice!). It's about getting our weight to where we want it to be, so we feel good about ourselves and remain healthy and active.

Why is midlife weight loss so hard?

Midlife is generally thought to begin at the age of 40 and spans the next 20 years of life. However, the physiological changes associated with midlife can begin earlier than this and, depending on how well we age (a result of both genetic and lifestyle factors), we can stay fit, healthy and active well beyond 60.

So, does it really get harder to manage our weight as we get older? What's the explanation for the spare tyre that appears as if from nowhere and attaches itself stubbornly around our middle? And why is it so damn hard to shift? If you've tried to lose weight after 40 but given up after seeing little reward for your efforts, you are not alone. Midlife weight loss can feel like mission impossible.

It may come as a relief to know that you are *not* imagining it. The changes we undergo in midlife do have an impact on our waistline; it's not simply overindulgence or a lack of dieting willpower that is causing the scales to head north. There are some specific reasons for putting on weight in our middle years, and we need to understand what's happening in our bodies before we attempt to address it. Let's start with our hormones.

HORMONES

Of all the changes our bodies undergo in midlife, the decline in hormone production (progesterone and oestrogen for women, testosterone for men) is perhaps the most profound. This process can begin as soon as our late thirties. It affects not just body fat distribution but can also lead to disrupted sleep, lower energy levels and mood swings, which in turn affect our eating patterns.

Women

So how does decreasing hormone production impact our weight in midlife? A comprehensive review by the International Menopause Society found that, contrary to popular belief, going through the menopause does not in itself cause women to gain weight – but it does lead to a change in the way that fat is distributed. According to review leader Professor Susan Davis from Monash University in Australia:

> It is a myth that the menopause causes a woman to gain weight. It's really just a consequence of environmental factors and ageing which cause that. But there is no doubt that the new spare tyre many women complain of after menopause is real, and not a consequence of any changes they have made. Rather, this is the body's response to the fall in oestrogen at menopause: a shift of fat storage from the hips to the waist.[9]

I spoke to Dr Louise Newson, a GP and menopause specialist based in Stratford-upon-Avon, who explained further:

> There are various reasons why women often put on weight during their perimenopause and menopause. The low oestrogen levels that occur lead to metabolic changes in our bodies. I see and speak to so many women who tell me they are comfort-eating to try and improve the way they feel. Low oestrogen levels that occur during the perimenopause and menopause can lead to sugar cravings and increased hunger, which can be hard to ignore. Also, women who are tired, low in their mood, anxious, or have reduced concentration and are less interested in life tend to eat a worse diet. It can be very difficult to be motivated to eat a good diet when hormone levels are reduced.[10]

In summary, hormonal changes in midlife, while perhaps not directly responsible for weight gain, can lead to a redistribution of fat around our waists. Also, the physiological effects of these hormonal changes can make us more susceptible to putting on weight: if we are tired, achy, have low energy and generally feel down in the dumps, we are less predisposed to exercise, or we may reach for food as a form of comfort.

Men

Men may also experience weight gain in midlife, but whereas women report a more general 'middle-aged spread', men are far more likely to accumulate fat up front – the classic D-shaped belly. This is a particular cause for concern because, regardless of your overall weight, having a large amount of belly fat (or visceral fat, as it's known) increases your risk of a range of diseases, such as cardiovascular disease, Type 2 diabetes and colorectal cancer.[11]

The underlying cause of these physiological changes in male body shape is not fully understood, but some studies suggest that declining testosterone – or what's known as the 'male menopause' – may be the reason. Testosterone production peaks for men in their late twenties. When they hit 30, it begins to decline by about 1% a year. It's estimated that as many as 10% of men aged 40 to 60 have low testosterone.[12] Now, that doesn't mean that they will all experience symptoms, but as Jeff Foster, a Warwickshire GP with an interest in men's health, explains: 'If you are struggling with weight gain despite working hard at the gym, if you have unexplained mood swings, fatigue and decreased libido it may be that deficient levels of testosterone are to blame. Improving your overall health by eating a healthy balanced diet, staying active and reducing stress can help support testosterone levels.'[13]

Can hormone replacement therapies help with weight management?

Dr Louise Newson advises that having body identical (that is, where the hormones given are chemically identical to those our bodies produce naturally) hormone replacement therapy (HRT) with oestrogen administered through the skin via a patch or gel often leads to weight loss. Some of this is because our hormones are being replaced, so the associated metabolic changes are lessened. In addition, women tend to feel better when they take HRT so are more likely to exercise and less likely to eat unhealthily.

Some of the synthetic progestogens in HRT can lead to fluid retention and even weight gain, however, so if a woman has put on weight with HRT then it is worth considering another type of HRT.

For men, there is the option of testosterone replacement therapy (TRT), a medical treatment that restores testosterone levels to the optimal physiological range. This can be administered in gel form or by injection.

Can what we eat affect our hormones?

There is no one food or supplement that can balance your hormones. The best advice is to eat a healthy, balanced diet; however, there are some foods that are thought to be particularly beneficial.

For women

- Broccoli: Cruciferous vegetables such as broccoli, Brussels sprouts, cabbage, cauliflower, kale, mustard greens and watercress contain the phytochemical indole-3-carbinol (I3C) which increases oestrogen metabolism.[14]
- Soy: Soybeans, edamame, tempeh and tofu are rich in isoflavones, a type of phytoestrogen. Phytoestrogens are chemicals produced by plants: they act like oestrogens in the body and are thought to lower rates of certain cancers, cardiovascular problems and menopausal symptoms.[15]

Introduction

Dr Jeff Foster cautions that TRT does not work for everyone; some men only see a small improvement in their symptoms. However, for most, when combined with lifestyle changes, the benefits may include less fat build-up, increased muscle mass and a better quality of sleep. At present TRT is only available on a restricted basis on the NHS but there are an increasing number of private clinics offering the treatment.

Some women also benefit from taking testosterone, which is another natural hormone produced by the ovaries. Testosterone therapy does not tend to lead to weight gain, and some women find they actually lose weight when using it.

- **Flax seeds:** Flax seeds are a good source of phytoestrogens, which can help to regulate levels of oestrogen in the body.
- **Avocado:** Avocado contains beneficial long chain fatty acids, which are crucial elements for hormonal production and function. Other sources of healthy fat are olive oil, nuts, seeds and oily fish.

For men

Vitamin D and zinc are both important for the production of testosterone.

- **Foods rich in vitamin D:** Oily fish such as trout, mackerel and salmon, foods fortified with vitamin D (e.g. milk and cereal) and egg yolks.
- **Foods rich in zinc:** Shellfish (especially oysters), beef, chicken, tofu, pork, nuts, seeds, lentils, yogurt, oats and mushrooms.

If you're considering taking either HRT or TRT, it's important to speak to your GP first to see if the treatment is appropriate for you.

What is clear from the current evidence is that declining hormones play a central role in weight gain and fat redistribution as we get older, but there are other age-related changes that can also make weight loss a challenge. Let's have a look at what happens to our metabolism in midlife.

METABOLISM

What is metabolism?

Put simply, metabolism is the chemical processes that occur within a living organism to maintain life. Our metabolism runs continuously to keep our bodies functioning, even when we are sleeping, by converting the food and nutrients we consume into the energy required to perform all our bodily functions: breathing, blood circulation, growing and repairing cells, and the elimination of waste.

The energy contained in our food is often expressed as calories (strictly speaking, kilocalories). We use the bulk of those calories (60–75%) just staying alive. This baseline of calorie expenditure is known as our *basal metabolic rate (BMR)* and it is determined by genetics, gender, height, weight, muscle mass and, of course, age. The other 25–40% of our daily caloric intake is used up by talking, walking, eating, digesting, exercising and even just thinking.

Does our metabolism change as we age?

Yes, indeed – our BMR begins to slow from about the age of 20. At first the decline is relatively slow and steady, at about 1–2% per decade, but after the age of 40 (in men) and 50 (in women), that rate of decline accelerates.[16] According to research carried out at Johns Hopkins University in the USA, that means that, in the absence of any lifestyle changes, the average adult will gain 1 to 2 pounds (about 0.5–1kg) per year from early adulthood through middle age.[17]

In the UK, Public Health England (PHE) currently recommends a daily calorie allowance of 2,500 for men and 2,000 for women.[18] However, even PHE thinks these figures are a bit on the generous side: it recently suggested that we could all do with eating 200–300 fewer calories per day.[19]

If you add this to the evidence of our slowing BMRs, we can see that if we want to keep our weight under control, our daily calorie intake in midlife should be around 1,600 for women and 2,000 for men. This will vary somewhat depending on activity levels, but it's easy to see how a muffin here and a latte there can easily blow our calorie budget.

Why does this slowdown happen?

There are three main factors that contribute to a slowing metabolism as we age: sarcopenia (or loss of muscle mass), decreasing physical activity and lipid turnover. Let's have a look at each of these in turn.

Muscle mass/sarcopenia

The biggest single determinant of a person's metabolism is lean mass: in other words, every part of our body that isn't fat, including our organs, blood vessels, skin, bones, water and, most importantly, muscle tissue.

Sarcopenia is the term given to age-related loss of muscle mass. The causes of sarcopenia are not fully understood but it is thought to be a combination of changes in hormones, immobility, age-related muscle changes, nutrition and neurodegenerative changes.[20]

Even if you are active, you'll still experience some muscle loss, but this is generally more pronounced in physically inactive people, who can lose as much as 3–5% of their muscle mass each decade after the age of 30.[21] The reason this matters when it comes to weight loss is that, the less muscle you have, the fewer calories you burn, which further slows your BMR.

And if you are male there's some more bad news, I'm afraid. Men's muscle mass declines even more sharply than women's in middle age, because of diminishing testosterone levels.[22] It is not known whether this in itself leads to a loss of muscle mass, but it is certainly a factor in muscle protein synthesis.[23]

Decreasing physical activity

Ageing is also associated with a decrease in physical activity, which may be gradual and therefore not easily perceived by an individual. There are various reasons why we tend to exercise less – or at least less vigorously – as we age, one of which is our innate capacity for exercise.

In a major study of more than 800 men and women aged 21 to 87 over a period of nearly eight years, researchers measured the decline in maximum exercise capacity as indicated by the amount of oxygen the body consumes during peak exercise performance. The results showed that aerobic capacity declined by 3–6% each decade in our twenties and thirties, but after the age of 70, the rate of decline accelerated to more than 20% per decade. The study also showed that after the age of 40, men's fitness levels declined at a faster rate than women, regardless of their level of physical activity.[24]

As exercise capacity declines, functional capacity (strength, endurance, agility and flexibility) levels also tend to reduce, which makes exercising harder and may discourage people further.

Any decrease in physical activity further accelerates age-related loss of muscle mass, leading to a further lowering of BMR – and so it goes on. Unless something is done to break this negative cycle, then health and fitness can quickly deteriorate.

Lipid turnover

Recent research has uncovered another reason for metabolic changes linked to ageing. A 2019 study carried out at the Karolinska Institutet in Sweden looked at the relationship between lipids (fat) and our metabolic system.[25] The research found that our lipid turnover – the rate at which we store and remove fat from our fat cells – slows down with age, causing weight gain due to a higher rate of fat storage.

In this trial, the Swedish team followed a group of 54 men and women for an average of thirteen years, and another group of

Can certain foods boost your metabolism?

When people talk about 'boosting their metabolism' what they really mean is increasing their BMR, or the number of calories they burn per day by doing nothing but existing.

While some studies have shown that certain foods, such as coffee, chilli and green tea, can have a temporary positive impact on our metabolism, this is nowhere near pronounced enough to contribute to weight loss.[26]

My advice is to eat or drink these things if you like the taste of them – but don't expect them to have any weight-loss benefits. The best way to support your metabolism is to eat a healthy, varied and balanced diet which will keep it functioning optimally.

41 women who had been morbidly obese before undergoing gastric band surgery, who were tracked for five years. In all of the participants, fat turnover slowed as they got to middle age and older, although not all gained weight.

Among those who did more exercise and consumed fewer calories, some maintained their weight, but participants who made no lifestyle changes and whose food intake, dietary composition and physical activities remained the same (or worsened) were found to have gained 20% of their body weight over the duration of the study: 'The results indicate for the first time that processes in our fat tissue regulate changes in body weight during ageing in a way that is independent of other factors,' said Peter Arner, the study's lead author.[27]

What this means is that weight gain in middle age is more or less inevitable unless we act to prevent it.

GUT HEALTH

So, we've seen how changes in our hormone levels and metabolism can affect our weight as we get older, but what about gut health? Does it have a part to play in midlife weight management?

What do we mean by gut health?

The human body is host to a vast number of microbes which together constitute what is known as our microbiota. Most of these reside in our small intestine and colon (the microbiome), and are essential to many aspects of our health and well-being. Gut microbes perform a number of functions: as well as absorbing energy and nutrients from our food, they can also influence our food cravings and play a role in signalling when we are full.

While there is no official definition of what constitutes a 'healthy gut', there are certain attributes of the microbiome that are associated with good gut health:

- **Richness/diversity:** Richness refers to the total number of bacterial species present in the gut microbiome, and diversity is the number of individual bacteria from each of the bacterial species.

- **Stability:** A stable microbiome is one that is resistant to factors that can potentially disrupt the microbiota. These include genetic factors, dietary modifications, age and various medications.

- **Resilience:** A resilient microbiome quickly returns to a healthy state after a disturbance – for example, after taking a course of antibiotics.

What role does our gut play in weight management?

Evidence is emerging that our microbiome plays a role in regulating body weight and as such is intrinsically linked to our obesity risk. A 2017 study by the National Institutes of Health (NIH),[28] one of the world's foremost medical research centres, found that our microbiota can affect both sides of the energy balance equation: first, as a factor influencing the amount of energy from food that we burn and, second, as a factor regulating the amount of energy we store.

Given that the composition of our microbiome is not fixed and can be influenced by dietary interventions, it's entirely possible that improving a person's diet could facilitate weight loss and prevent obesity.

What happens to our gut health as we age?

Many lifestyle and environmental factors contribute to our gut health, but what we are now beginning to understand is that age is also a factor.

More tips for better gut health

1. Eat a diet rich in fibre: Eat plenty of fruit, vegetables, whole grains and legumes. It's best to gradually increase fibre intake and drink plenty of water to enable the fibre to do its work.
2. Try fermented foods with probiotics: Some foods, such as live yogurt (I use this a lot in my recipes), naturally contain good bacteria. Other examples are miso, kefir, kimchi and kombucha.
3. Chew food well: Digestion starts in the mouth: chewing food properly is an important part of the digestive process.
4. Drink alcohol and caffeine in moderation: Alcohol can irritate the digestive tract and alter the bacterial balance of the gut. Caffeine causes a temporary increase in stress hormones, which is useful if you need a boost in the morning but may not be a good choice if you already feel stressed.
5. De-stress and sleep well: There's a direct link between the brain and gut, called the gut–brain axis, so being stressed and tired can profoundly affect gut health.
6. Exercise regularly: Exercise helps to regulate bowel movements and so is particularly helpful for those prone to constipation. It's also associated with greater microbial diversity.
7. Avoid unnecessary medications: Certain types of painkiller and antibiotic can aggravate gut problems and disrupt the gut microbiota, but of course sometimes they are necessary. After a course of antibiotics, it's even more important to replenish the microbiome by eating plenty of gut-friendly foods.

> 8. **Stop smoking:** Smoking is not only terrible for
>   your general health, but it also adversely affects gut
>   bacteria. It goes without saying that continuing to
>   smoke in midlife is a huge health no-no.
>
> For more advice on exercise, sleep, stress and alcohol reduc-
> tion, see the Midlife Method Healthy Habits on p. 52.

Researchers studying the gut bacteria of thousands of people across the globe have come to the conclusion that the microbiome is a surprisingly accurate biological clock, able to assess the age of most people to within a few years.[29] In the study, a team from InSilico Medicine, a US biotechnology company, examined more than 3,600 samples of gut bacteria from 1,165 healthy individuals from around the world. What they discovered was that some microbes became more abundant as people aged, such as *Eubacterium hallii*, which is important for certain metabolic processes in the gut. Others decreased, such as *Bacteroides vulgatus*, which has been linked to ulcerative colitis, a type of inflammation in the digestive tract.

This indicates that age does affect the make-up of the microbiome. While this in and of itself doesn't necessarily have implications for weight management, what we do know is that gut *diversity* is an important factor.

Another large-scale study looked into the relationship of age to gut bacterial diversity in adults from the USA, UK, Colombia and China.[30] Overall gut microbiome diversity correlated positively with age in young adults – in other words, it got more diverse with age – but tailed off around the age of 40 with no positive correlation in middle-aged adults.

In addition to compositional shifts, evidence is also gathering that our gut diversity, and consequently the efficiency with which we digest and metabolise food, declines after the age of 40. There may also be a gradual reduction in the production of gastric, pancreatic and other digestive secretions that are all crucial components of a healthy digestive system which in turn can lead to lower absorption of nutrients.[31]

What can we do to improve our gut health?

As we can see, supporting our gut health is crucially important as we get older, not just in terms of our general health, but also as a factor in weight management. A diet consisting of a wide variety of nutrient-dense foods is the key to maintaining a diverse gut microbiome. Dr Megan Rossi, better known as the Gut Health Doctor and author of the excellent book *Eat Yourself Healthy*, advises:

> The first thing to realise is that you need to eat as wide a range of plant-based foods as possible. I advise people to aim for 30 different plant-based foods – that's nuts, seeds, whole grains, legumes, and fruit and veggies – a week. Research has suggested that if you are having less than ten of these plant-based foods a week, your microbial diversity isn't very strong. Try to vary the foods you eat from week to week, and always be open to trying new things.[32]

The Midlife Method places whole, plant-based foods at the heart of its approach to healthy eating, including plenty of healthy fats, good-quality lean protein and complex carbohydrates for optimum nutrition. Since a healthy microbiome is key to supporting our weight-loss efforts, we need to ensure that what we are eating, while still low enough in calories to achieve that all-important energy deficit, is not deficient when it comes to our gut health.

Now we understand what's going on in these midlife bodies of ours, let's move on to what we are going to do to lose weight and feel great.

The Midlife Method

The Midlife Method is not a diet in the sense that it will begin and end. The Four-Week Meal Plan in this book is just the start: it is designed to help us reprogramme how we think about food and what we eat. We are aiming for long-term change that will, over time, enable us to reach a healthy, maintainable body weight.

Research undertaken by Tufts University in the USA[33] has shown that the brain can effectively be retrained to prefer healthy food. The study focused on changing food preferences by prescribing a diet higher in fibre and protein, and lower in carbohydrates, but which did not allow participants to become hungry (because that is when food cravings take over and unhealthy food becomes attractive).

Alarm bells might be ringing about now – perhaps you're already worried about having to live off boring salads or having to stop eating your favourite foods altogether (No more croissants! Cheese! Wine!). Don't worry; no foods are absolutely off-limits. The aim is to calorie-restrict enough to enable weight loss while rebalancing your diet to ensure good nutrition. The focus is on enjoying food more, not less.

The other stumbling block for many people when trying to make dietary changes is how to feed their family at the same time without having to make multiple different meals. Wherever possible, I have designed the recipes to be family-friendly or have added tips so you can adjust them to suit your family's likes and dislikes.

How it works

As we have discovered, there are a number of things working against us that can make weight management in midlife a challenge: declining hormones, a slowing metabolism and a less efficient digestive system. The Midlife Method, therefore, is a holistic, three-pronged plan for addressing these issues to lose weight and feel great. It comprises the following:

Light Days: On Light Days the focus is on achieving an energy deficit for weight loss by sticking to an 800-calorie limit. The number of Light Days you do per week depends on the amount of weight you wish to lose, and how quickly. A minimum of three Light Days a week is required to see some progress: however, the Four-Week Meal Plan included later in the book starts with six Light Days in the first week, while motivation is high, to achieve a rapid initial weight loss. The number of Light Days is then reduced gradually to three per week by Week 4. This is continued until you reach your target weight.

Regular Days: On Regular Days the focus is not on calorie restriction but on eating balanced, nutrient-dense food to ensure adequate nutrition and a healthy gut. Having said that, it is important to stick to a rough allowance of 1,600 calories for a woman or 2,000 for a man so you don't undo all the good work done on Light Days.

The Midlife Method Healthy Habits: Exercise, decent sleep, stress management, alcohol moderation – all are critical pieces of the midlife health jigsaw puzzle to support your metabolism and physical well-being. The Midlife Method Healthy Habits will provide all the information and knowledge you need to make positive changes in these areas, enhancing your weight-loss efforts.

LIGHT DAYS

As we have discussed, the key to weight loss is maintaining an energy deficit over a sustained period of time: in other words, our total energy intake needs to be less than our total energy expenditure. The most effective way to achieve this deficit is via what we eat.

Of course, exercise uses up energy so it certainly has a role to play, but to put it in context, we'd have to do 272 burpees to burn off one slice of pepperoni pizza (260 calories); it's far, far easier to manage our weight by adjusting what we eat. As the saying goes, you can't exercise your way out of a poor diet, although exercise is important for all sorts of reasons, which we will cover later on.

I am absolutely sure that if you've dieted in the past you will have very negative associations around calorie restriction. You were probably not eating foods you liked or enjoyed, they probably weren't filling, so you felt hungry a lot of the time, and perhaps you felt like you were constantly having to 'be good', saying no to all the things you love to eat?

If so, you're not alone. This is the way most diets make us feel, and is ultimately why they fail. The question is, how can we make calorie restriction do-able? The answer is to focus on calorie restriction *just a few days a week* so it's not too onerous and it gives us enough flexibility to live our lives. I call these Light Days.

On a Light Day we aim to eat a total of 800 calories, which can be distributed however you wish throughout the day. I generally opt for a calorie split roughly 200/300/300 between my three meals, although this can vary depending on what I'm doing that day. Avoid snacking on a Light Day, and stick to water, tea or coffee (with a splash of milk, if you like) for drinks.

How many Light Days do we need to do each week for weight loss?

This depends on how quickly you want to lose weight. As mentioned previously, a minimum of three Light Days per week is required to see any tangible results but, since we tend to be more highly motivated at the beginning of any new regime, it makes sense to try and do more Light Days initially to see quick results. Studies have found that participants in weight-loss programmes are dependent on weight loss for continuing to invest in the process:[34] in other words, the more quickly we see results, the more motivated we are to continue.

My Four-Week Meal Plan, therefore, front-loads the Light Days so you start off doing more Light Days. They then gradually decrease over the four weeks:

- Week 1: six Light Days/one Regular Day
- Week 2: five Light Days/two Regular Days
- Week 3: four Light Days/three Regular Days
- Week 4: three Light Days/four Regular Days.

If, at the end of the four weeks, you still have more weight to lose, you can continue with three Light Days a week until you reach your goal. To maintain your weight, it's enough to do one or two Light Days a week.

You might be wondering how this plan differs from intermittent fasting diets such as the 5:2 and the Fast 800 diet, which also advocate calorie-restricting a few days a week. In truth, they have a lot in common, but the main difference is that, with the Midlife Method, *when* you eat is totally up to you; there are no time restrictions or set fasting windows.

Tips to make Light Days a doddle

All the recipes in this book are designed to make it easy to stick to the 800-calorie count, but here are some general tips for making Light Days a doddle.

Be organised: Plan your meals in advance and make sure you have the right ingredients to hand so you don't get derailed.

Have the right kit: You don't need a load of specialist kit, but it is worth investing in a decent set of scales, a food processor for chopping and blending, a hand mixer for mixing and whisking, and a good non-stick frying pan to minimise the amount of oil you use when cooking.

Leftovers are king. If you are making a recipe, why not make double so you can have some for the next day? As one of my Instagram followers said, leftovers are money in the bank. I couldn't agree more!

Batch-cook and freeze. Plenty of the recipes in this book can be made in larger quantities so you can freeze them for a later date.

Focus on flavour. If you wish to try out your own creations, focus on ingredients that pack a low-calorie flavour hit, such as chilli, soy, lemon, ginger, garlic, fresh herbs and spices.

Hydrate. Drink lots of water and herbal tea, or try keeping a jug of unsweetened iced tea with fresh ginger in the fridge.

Of course, there has been much scientific study into the health benefits of fasting, and it may be something you are keen to incorporate, so you can if you so choose. You could divide your 800 calories between breakfast and dinner, or skip breakfast and divide the calories between lunch and dinner. It's up to you. If I skip a meal then I feel absolutely ravenous as the day progresses and I'm far more likely to make poor food choices, but we are all different.

In addition, the Midlife Method is flexible: you can adjust the number of Light Days to suit your ability to calorie-restrict, so if you feel that starting Week 1 with six Light Days is too much (although you might surprise yourself!), you can just do three or four Light Days from the start. You should still see results; it will just take a little longer to reach your target weight.

See Light Days as a tool for you to use in a way that is appropriate to your weight-loss needs.

REGULAR DAYS

While Light Days are concerned with calorie restriction, on Regular Days the focus shifts to eating a healthy, well-balanced diet. Having said that, it is still important to keep an eye on how much you are eating and stick to the suggested calorie allowance of 1,600 calories for a woman and 2,000 for a man (or your own personal Regular Day calorie allowance – see below), otherwise you risk negating the weight loss progress made on Light Days.

The meal plans in this book are designed to fit with this calorie allowance. Since you have a few more calories to play with on Regular Days than on Light Days, you can afford to have the odd snack, healthy treat or perhaps even a glass of wine in the evening.

Calculating your Regular Day calorie allowance

For most 'average' midlifers (a person aged between 40 and 60, who exercises regularly and with no underlying medical conditions) a calorie allowance of 1,600 per day for a woman and 2,000 per day for a man is about right: not so high that we risk putting on weight, not so low that we don't have enough energy to function optimally.

However, your circumstances may mean a different Regular Day calorie allowance is appropriate. You may, for example, be extremely active or have a physically demanding job. If this is the case, you can set a Regular Day calorie allowance that is personal to you. There are many calorie calculators on the internet to use to do this – I have included a good one in the Resources at the end of the book.

The Midlife Method 'Regular Day' Toolkit

So, Regular Days are all about eating for overall good health, discovering nutrient-dense foods that you love, and learning to handle food cravings so you ultimately make better food choices.

To help you do this, I have created the Midlife Method 'Regular Day' Toolkit which comprises five practical techniques to help you eat well on Regular Days. They are:

1. Eat with awareness.

2. Eat mainly nutrifoods.

3. Be calorie-aware.

4. Mind the macros.

5. Practise volume control.

Let's have a look at each of these tools and see how they can help us make better food choices.

Eat with awareness

Now you're probably thinking that 'eating with awareness' sounds an awful lot like 'mindful eating', which is a term that has been bandied about a lot in recent years. Mindful eating may have 'woo' connotations, but what exactly is it and how can it help us?

Mindfulness has its roots in Buddhism, but it is something we can all access. 'Mindfulness means awareness – an innate quality that we all have but gets easily lost in the rush of life,' explains Professor Mark Williams, Professor of Clinical Psychology at the University of Oxford and the author of several books on mindfulness. 'One way to understand it is to think of its opposite: "mindlessness" – when we aren't really aware of what we are doing from one moment to another. It means that life is not enjoyed as much as it could be.'[35]

Once you reframe 'mindful eating' as 'eating with awareness', it makes a lot more sense, and it's immediately obvious that being more aware of what you eat is the key to a better relationship with food. Rather than mindlessly grabbing a takeaway meal or a snack, our enjoyment of eating is enhanced when we eat tasty food that is also providing our body with what it needs to thrive.

In practice, eating with awareness is about giving ourselves permission to eat well, to take the time needed to make conscious food choices, and to enjoy the act of eating. To get started, try asking yourself these questions every time you feel like eating something:

- Why do I want to eat right now?
- How hungry am I on a scale of 1 to 10?
- Will this food be delicious and worth eating?
- How will I feel after I eat it?
- Does it taste good enough for me to carry on eating it?

- Have I had enough now?
- How satisfied do I feel on a scale of 1 to 10?

After a while you won't need to ask yourself these questions consciously; you will instinctively know what, when and how much to eat. Even when choosing to eat something for pleasure, you will be able to do so without judgement.

That's the beauty of eating with awareness: it can help you make better food choices but it can also help you lose any guilt you might feel around eating something that isn't, strictly speaking, 'good for you'. You can give yourself permission, from time to time, to eat something purely because you enjoy eating it.

While eating with awareness is primarily concerned with eating well on Regular Days, it can also help support weight loss. By being more aware of what you eat, you will make better food choices – and this, on its own, should have an impact on your waistline.

However, there are specific areas that can help to accelerate weight loss if that is your aim:

- **Minimise calorific foods with little nutritional value.** A large part of eating with awareness is recognising the difference between hunger and cravings. Cravings generally involve foods that are high in calories but low in nutritional value. Try to find healthy foods you really love to eat.

- **Capitalise on those days when you don't feel hungry.** Some days you'll be ravenous; on other days you'll hardly think of food at all. Tune in to your body's natural appetite and eat accordingly.

- **Be aware of your portion size.** This is a quick win if your eyes tend to be bigger than your stomach. Only eat what you need to feel full.

- **Keep hydrated.** Thirst and hunger are easily confused. If you feel peckish, have a drink of water and see if that does the trick.

When it comes to mealtimes, there are some other things to consider when eating with awareness:

1. **Am I overdoing the extras?**
   For example, if you usually have a sandwich, a bag of crisps and a piece of fruit for lunch, what about dropping the crisps? It's probably just a habit you've got into and the crisps don't deliver anything nutritionally.

2. **Am I adding calories unnecessarily?**
   For example, if you have a jacket potato for lunch, instead of loading it with butter and cheese, why not swap these for a mixture of Greek yogurt and chopped spring onion instead? Fewer calories and still delicious.

3. **What does my body need from this meal?**
   How balanced have your meals been today? Have you had enough lean protein? Enough fruit and veg? Enough complex carbs? There's no need to overcomplicate things, but if you had a jacket potato earlier then focus on more protein and veg at dinner time.

4. **What if I've exercised?**
   If you've exercised in the morning, a lunch with plenty of good fats and protein will help your recovery. A mixed leaf salad with a few slices of avocado, some cooked chicken and an olive oil-based dressing would be ideal.

5. **Can I have dessert?**
   Yes, but favour fruit. It is worth investing in a ready supply of your favourite fruits. Most desserts are full of calories and low in nutrition. Although they're not off-limits, they should be kept for special occasions.

As you can see from these examples, eating with awareness isn't about *not* eating; it is about being conscious of what your body needs and eating accordingly. Rather than the traditional diet mindset of 'I must not eat X – it's bad', you can reframe it and think instead 'My body does not *need* X; maybe I'll have Y instead' (Y being a more nutritious food choice). It's very liberating to think about food this way; not in terms of what we *cannot* eat but in terms of what we *can* eat to nourish our bodies and feel satisfied.

Eating with awareness is at the heart of the Midlife Method. Not only will it transform your relationship with food, but it is also key to long-term weight management.

Eat mainly nutrifoods

So here it is, the inevitable truth. If we want to lose weight and be healthier, we have to make good food choices. It's not exactly earth-shattering news, I'm not telling you anything you don't already know, but sometimes it's just not that easy making it happen in real life.

It all sounds fine in theory – eat more oily fish, veg, nuts, seeds, etc. – but that doesn't always translate to what ends up in the shopping trolley. This week, as an exercise, have a look at how much of your usual weekly food shop comprises what I call nutrifoods. Nutrifoods are foods that:

- are high in nutritional value (for example, brightly coloured fruit and veg, nuts, seeds, eggs, whole grains, lean protein such as fish, chicken, etc.)
- are minimally processed (so a block of cheese is fine but cheese strings, not so much!)
- have no artificial colours, flavours, preservatives or unrecognisable ingredients.

You might be surprised at how much of what you buy is processed: jars of sauce or marinades, bottled salad dressings, boxes of fishcakes, an 'emergency' frozen pizza, packet cereals (even the 'good' ones are usually high in sugar), sausages, a regular sliced loaf, etc.

Processed foods can contain high levels of simple carbohydrates (sugar) and saturated fat, so it is harder to ensure we are eating a balanced diet when they are the mainstay of our food intake.

Here's a quick summary:

Nutrifoods – consume most of the time	**Not so nutritious – OK occasionally**
Fresh (preferably organic or free-range) meat and chicken	Processed meat and meat products (bacon, ham, burgers, sausages, etc.)
Fresh fish and seafood	Shop-bought fishcakes or crumbed/battered fillets
Freshly baked wholegrain bread	Regular sliced loaves
Wholemeal pittas or wraps	Crumpets, plain bagels, muffins
Fresh fruit	Juices and fruit drinks
Olive oil	Butter
Eggs	Shop-bought mayonnaise
Homemade porridge	Shop-bought porridge mixes
Sugar-free muesli/granola (or make your own: see My Go-to Granola, p. 89)	Most other packet cereals
Raw nuts and seeds	Cereal or granola bars
Wholegrain pasta	White pasta
Brown rice	White rice
Quinoa or bulgur wheat	Regular couscous (choose wholegrain)

The table above illustrates how a few good shopping choices can have a big impact on the quality of your diet. So next time you pick up something processed at the supermarket, think about whether there might be a better nutrifood alternative.

Now your cupboards are stocked with nutrifoods, it's much easier to make meals from scratch and cut down on the processed versions.

> **Example:** Pasta and a ready-made sauce was always my fall-back family dinner on busy days, but it wasn't really such a healthy meal. White pasta is a simple carbohydrate and low in fibre, and shop-bought pasta sauce can contain lots of salt and sugar. What to do? I found a good wholegrain pasta (which didn't taste of cardboard!) and I made a load of my own Rich Tomato Sauce (see p. 128) which I froze in meal-sized portions. It can easily be jazzed up with fresh veg, olives, prawns, fresh herbs or chilli.

A final word on nutrifoods – please remember that nothing is completely off-limits. Denying ourselves the things we love to eat is unsustainable; the aim is to gently move away from eating processed/convenience foods towards eating mainly nutritious, unprocessed food. So, if on a Regular Day you fancy something that is not right at the top of the nutritional league table, that's fine. Just don't go mad. Moderation is the name of the game.

Be calorie-aware

While rigorous calorie counting is undoubtedly a chore, the only proven way to lose weight is to achieve an energy deficit. To do that, we need to have a rough idea of our calorie intake. The Midlife Method makes this easy because the majority of the calorie restriction is taken care of on our Light Days, which means we can be more relaxed on Regular Days. However, we do still need to be aware of the calories we are consuming so as not to blow our Light Day efforts.

Calorie awareness means having a sense of the relative calorie loads of different foods, even those that are healthy. I meet so many frustrated people who insist they eat healthily but can't shift any weight. It's perfectly possible to 'eat well' and put on weight. Why? Because some healthy foods are surprisingly calorific, such as avocados, nuts and nut butters, granola, energy balls and vegan desserts, which often include lots of nuts, seeds and oil.

Example: A good friend of mine was getting very frustrated with her inability to lose weight. On one of our morning walks, I quizzed her about her typical daily food intake. She had switched to snacking on nuts because they were healthier, but it turns out she was working her way through a large bag of almonds every day: 100g of almonds has 636 calories! A snack-size portion of almonds is around thirteen nuts or 100 calories.

How to snack well

Tuning in to our body's hunger signals is really important if we want to manage our weight effectively, so next time you feel hungry, ask yourself these questions (this is eating with awareness in action):

1. Am I genuinely hungry? On a scale of 1 to 10, if it's less than 8 you probably don't need a snack.
2. Am I just bored or do I need a break? Maybe go for a walk, stretch, have a cup of tea.
3. Am I thirsty? Thirst and hunger are often confused. Have a big glass of water and see if that helps.
4. Can I ride it out until the next meal? If it's not far off, resist munching for the sake of it.

Here are some tasty nutrifood snacks all under 100 calories:

- two tablespoons of Greek yogurt with a handful of raspberries
- an oatcake or wholegrain cracker with a dried fig

Now, I'm not suggesting we stop eating healthy foods because they are calorific; we just need to keep an eye on the quantity. Similarly, we don't need to be calorie-counting experts to be calorie-aware, it's mainly common sense:

> **Example:** I'm meeting a friend at a local coffee shop. I could have a white Americano or a flat white. Both are coffees with milk but because I am being calorie-aware I know that the white Americano only contains a splash of milk. The flat white is made predominantly from milk, so it's easy to see that the calorie count of the flat white is going to be higher. It doesn't really matter how many calories it has exactly, but I know enough to make the lower-calorie choice, so I go for the white Americano.

- a Medjool date with a teaspoon of nut butter
- a square of dark chocolate and a few salted peanuts
- an apple, pear, orange or small banana
- a small number of nuts (13 almonds is 100 calories)
- a crispbread cracker with a smearing of hummus
- some raw veggie sticks and one tablespoon of one of these easy homemade dips:

Carrot & Mint Dip: Two carrots peeled and steamed (or boiled) until very soft, one tablespoon of light cream cheese, a few sprigs of fresh mint, salt and pepper. Whizz in a food processor or blender.

Beetroot & Cumin Dip: Three cooked beetroots from a packet, one tablespoon of Greek yogurt, a pinch of ground cumin, a squeeze of lemon juice, salt and pepper. Whizz in a food processor or blender.

Yogurt & Cucumber Dip: 100g Greek yogurt, 10cm length cucumber (grated), a squeeze of lemon juice, salt and pepper. Mix the ingredients together in a bowl.

In actual fact, the calorie count is roughly:

White Americano, 25 cals   Flat white, 125 cals

Of course many of us (me included!) prefer a flat white, but if we just have one or two a week and stick to white Americanos the rest of the time, we can easily save a couple of hundred calories a day – that could be as much as 1,400 calories over the course of the week.

Healthy foods that are surprisingly high in calories

We all know the more unhealthy calorific foods that we should limit in our diet (cakes, crisps, biscuits, chips, pizza, butter, cream, etc.) but here are some healthy foods that are relatively high in calories and should be eaten in moderation:

- Nut butters – they have almost 100 calories per tablespoon.
- Tahini – delicious but calorific (about the same as nut butter).
- Bread – around 100 calories per slice. Choose wholegrain.
- Nuts, seeds, granola – excellent nutrient value but high in calories. Have just a few, or a light sprinkle.
- Olive oil – very nutritious, but drizzle it rather than slosh.
- Coconut milk – use the lighter version.
- Avocados – full of good fat. Stick to a portion size of one quarter of an avocado.
- Oily fish – one to two portions a week have excellent nutritional benefits, but white fish and shellfish are lower in calories.
- Dried fruit – very high in sugar, and bad for your teeth! Stick to fresh fruit.

Another way to think about managing calories is what I call food spend. On any given day, we have a certain number of calories we require for our body to function properly. We can eat this amount without weight gain being an issue. Eat over this amount and, unless we are doing a lot of physical activity, the extra calories or energy will be converted to fat and stored. As we start our day, and begin eating, we are using up that calorie allowance. This is our food spend.

Put another way, imagine you have £10 to spend on food for the day and no more. You would think carefully about the relative value of the food you were buying. Sticking with the coffee example, is it better to spend £5 on a flat white and a muffin or £2.50 on a white Americano and a banana? The second option is clearly preferable: cheaper and better for us nutritionally. This doesn't mean we can never eat a muffin again; it's just about shifting our focus, seeing the muffin as something to be enjoyed once in a while, eaten with awareness, and acknowledging that it's not something we should eat regularly if we're trying to lose weight.

There's quite a lot to digest there – no pun intended – but most of it is just good old-fashioned common sense. Nothing is off-limits; it's all about balance and proportion. Being calorie-aware is the key to weight management once you have reached your target weight.

Mind the macros

Macros, or macronutrients, are what make up the calorie content of food. When we talk about a 'balanced' diet, really what we mean is one that includes a balance of the three macronutrients: healthy fats, lean proteins and complex carbohydrates.

Let's look at each of the macronutrients in turn and see what they bring to the table.

Fat

For many years fat was the enemy, and low-fat diets were very popular. As a famous actress once said, 'If you don't eat fat you won't get fat' – reason enough not to take nutritional advice from celebrities!

What is true is that fat is more calorific than the other macro-nutrients – protein and carbohydrate contain just 4 calories per gram while fat has 9 – so eating less fat is an easy way to cut calories. However, we need some fat in our diet for all sorts of reasons, including brain development, hormone production and the absorption of the fat-soluble vitamins (A, D, E, K).

Good sources of fat include:

- avocados
- olives and olive oil
- dairy (milk, yogurt)
- nuts (almonds, walnuts, cashews)
- seeds (chia, pumpkin, flax)
- oily fish (sardines, mackerel, salmon, trout).

When adding fat during the cooking or food preparation process, use extra virgin olive oil (for dressings) or light olive oil/organic rapeseed oil (for cooking). By all means keep some proper butter in the fridge for when the occasion calls for it, but try to use it sparingly if you have a tendency to slather.

Protein

Protein provides amino acids, which are the building blocks of cell and muscle structure. There are 20 types of amino acid, nine of which are essential, meaning that your body must get them from food as the body cannot make them itself. Protein is not just important for maintaining muscle mass (especially crucial in later life); it is the core component of organs, bones, hair and enzymes. It also supports a healthy immune system.

Good sources of protein include:

- fish and seafood (salmon, tuna, white fish, shrimp, crab)
- poultry (chicken and turkey)
- lean meat (pork, beef, lamb)
- eggs
- dairy (cheese, unsweetened yogurt)
- tofu, tempeh and edamame
- legumes (beans, peas, chickpeas, lentils and peanuts)
- hemp and chia seeds
- quinoa.

Carbohydrate

The topic of carbs has been – if you'll excuse the pun – a hot potato in recent years, thanks to the popularity of low-carb diets. For a while it seemed that a good proportion of the population had simply stopped eating carbs: a triumph of marketing over nutritional common sense, you might say.

Yes, it's true that eating too many *simple* carbs (white pasta/bread/rice and processed foods with added sugars) can sabotage our efforts to lose weight and improve our health; conversely, however, eating a moderate amount of *complex* carbs can help in both these endeavours.

Complex carbs are key to maintaining energy levels, hormone balance, and a host of other important metabolic functions. Rather than cutting out carbs, we need to consider the amount and types of carbs we are eating. Western diets are skewed in favour of carbohydrates, so most of us can afford to cut down on the quantity of carbs we are eating in favour of lean protein and vegetables. Some carbohydrate is good; a whole plateful of rice, noodles or pasta is too much.

Good sources of complex carbohydrates include:

- whole grains (oats, quinoa, brown rice)
- wholegrain bread and pasta
- beans and legumes, including peas
- sweet potatoes and squash
- fresh fruit (especially apples, berries and bananas)
- vegetables (especially leafy greens, broccoli and carrots)
- nuts and seeds.

Macro balance

Much has been made of macro counting as a weight-management tool. While there is no evidence to support a 'perfect' split of macros, it is generally agreed that a good proportion of protein in the diet may be beneficial for these reasons:

1. **Satiety:** We tend to feel fuller after eating a protein-rich meal, leading to a reduction in our overall calorie intake.

2. **Thermic effect:** It takes more energy to metabolise and store protein than the other macronutrients, which may help increase our energy expenditure.

3. **Muscle mass:** Protein helps us retain lean muscle, which is important in supporting our BMR.

In summary, each of the three macronutrients is essential to good nutrition. While overall calorie intake has the biggest impact on weight loss, balancing macronutrients is key to ensuring the weight-loss process is healthy and sustainable. The acceptable macronutrient distribution range produced by the Food and Nutrition Board of the Institutes of Medicine gives the standard macro intake ranges as follows:[36]

- fat: 20–35% of calories

- protein: 10–35% of calories

- carbs: 45–65% of calories.

In midlife we benefit from getting a higher proportion of our calorie intake from lean protein and healthy fats and a little less from carbohydrates, so the daily meal combinations and weekly meal plans for the Midlife Method average out at around 30% fat, 25% protein and 45% carbohydrates.

Don't forget about fibre

Fibre is a type of carbohydrate that the body can't digest. As well as keeping our bowels functioning properly, fibre plays a role in weight management.

There are two ways that fibre helps to regulate our appetite. First, it makes us feel fuller for longer because it delays the emptying of food from the stomach. Second, it slows the absorption of glucose into the bloodstream, avoiding spikes in blood sugar. Keeping our blood sugar levels steady is important because sugar spikes are usually followed by hunger pangs as our blood sugar drops back down again.

This is particularly relevant in midlife. When we are rushed off our feet looking after our families, working long hours or simply trying to fit too many things into our day, we may well turn to sugary foods for an energy boost. But good hydration and eating more fibre are the best way to address this problem. So, next time you experience a sugar craving, have a big glass of water and a healthy fibre-rich snack instead (see How to snack well on p. 42).

Practise volume control

Another tool to help us avoid overeating on a Regular Day is to simply eat a bit less across the board, something I call *volume control*.

We tend to overeat by sheer force of habit, loading up our plate because it's what we've always done, but most people can eat 20% less than usual without noticing any difference in satiety levels. It's thought that our stomachs have an 'appetite thermostat' and can become accustomed to receiving a certain quantity of food. If we can slowly turn the thermostat down, we will feel satisfied by less food.[37]

On a practical level, here's how to get started with volume control:

- **Don't overload your plate.** Put a reasonable amount of food on your plate, eat it slowly, and only have more if you are still feeling hungry.

- **Having pasta?** Have a portion of pasta the size of your clenched fist with sauce, and fill the rest of the plate with salad or veg.

- **Having pizza?** Have one or two slices and fill the rest of your plate with salad or veg.

- **Having roast dinner?** Have fewer roast potatoes and less meat, have more veg. Go easy on the gravy.

- **Having curry?** Have a teacup-sized portion of curry, the same quantity of brown rice, and a load of chopped-up cucumber, tomato and plain yogurt.

- **Having a sandwich?** Maybe have an open sandwich to reduce the amount of bread, or choose a wholegrain wrap or use large romaine lettuce leaves as a wrap for the filling.

- **Try not to pick at leftovers.** When you're finished, clear the table straight away. In a restaurant, ask the waiter to remove half-empty plates.

Eating well on Regular Days isn't difficult, but it does require some focus. The Midlife Method 'Regular Day' Toolkit is a set of simple messages we can use to make better food choices. Just remember:

1. Eat with awareness.

2. Eat mainly nutrifoods.

3. Be calorie-aware.

4. Mind the macros.

5. Practise volume control.

The Midlife Method Healthy Habits:
exercise, sleep, stress, alcohol

Time for a recap. So far we've seen how, on Light Days, the focus is on weight loss via calorie restriction. On Regular Days the emphasis is on weight maintenance through good nutrition. And here's the final piece of the puzzle: the Midlife Method Healthy Habits. Making positive lifestyle changes not only supports our weight-loss efforts, but also helps us feel better both physically and mentally.

These are the four main areas of focus:

- exercise
- sleep
- stress
- alcohol.

EXERCISE

Why is exercise important in midlife?

Exercise is beneficial whatever our age, but as we move into our middle years it becomes even more important. Adding to the body of evidence that exercise can help midlife (and older) adults improve their longevity, a 2019 study[38] found that sedentary adults aged 40 to 80 who increased their physical activity level to 150 minutes a week were 24% less likely to die during the study period than those who remained inactive.

That's a pretty compelling statistic – and the good news is, it's never too late to begin. Even if you have been relatively inactive, taking up exercise in midlife can help improve blood pressure, blood sugar and cholesterol levels and reduce inflammation.

Exercise is something I came to relatively late in life. I have never loved exercise; I did very little at school, virtually none at university, and the odd reluctant step class in my twenties. As I got older it became more apparent that I had to make exercise a part of my life, and now I exercise most days. I still don't *love* exercise, but I have learned to love how it makes me feel.

Another barrier to exercising in midlife can be our increasingly achy bodies: joints can feel stiff in the morning and muscles tight and inflexible. Or we may have lingering injuries or other physical limitations that can hamper our efforts to stay fit. Don't use these as an excuse to remain inactive – most physical issues can be improved with the correct interventions, so go and see your doctor or a physical therapist who can get you up and running again – or at least brisk walking, if that's more your thing!

Can exercise help me to lose weight?

In terms of weight loss, exercise will of course burn some calories and, since weight loss is largely down to creating a calorie deficit (a fancy way of saying fewer calories in than out), then exercise is clearly part of that equation.

Let's think about this a bit more. How do food and exercise compare in the context of calories? Remember the example I gave earlier: that it takes 272 burpees to burn off one slice of pepperoni pizza (260 calories)? I was in two minds about giving this as an example because all too often exercise is used as a way to justify poor food choices – and in that sense it can be seen as a form of punishment. I prefer to focus on the health benefits that exercise confers, rather than thinking of it simply as a way to burn calories. The point of my example is to illustrate how it's far easier to control our energy balance through what we eat than try to exercise off any excess.

So, given that managing our weight is largely down to our food intake rather than how much we exercise, why is exercise such an important part of the Midlife Method? Well, it's back to that all-important BMR again.

Sustained calorie reduction can lead to a lowering of BMR, which somewhat negates the effect of reduced caloric intake. Exercise counters this by keeping the metabolism firing and maintaining muscle mass.

Even if you're not losing weight, regular physical activity can improve health markers such as insulin sensitivity, cholesterol levels and blood pressure, which lowers your risk of developing chronic illnesses later in life. So whichever way you cut it, exercise in midlife is essential.

How much exercise should I do? What types of exercise are best?

I'm sure you will have seen this among your own social circle, or perhaps even experienced it yourself: hitting midlife can elicit an extreme reaction – running a marathon, swimming an ocean or climbing a mountain. But before you sign up for that triathlon, note that there's increasing evidence that a more varied, moderate approach to exercise is better as we get older.

A study published by the journal *Circulation*[39] looked at the role of exercise in improving heart health in midlife. It found the optimal amount of exercise is four to five 30-minute sessions a week, including a mix of high- and low-intensity activity, strength/resistance training, and at least one longer session of aerobic exercise, such as an hour of tennis, cycling or running.

This might seem like a lot, but the aim is simply to be active most days. If you don't have time for a class, a quick walk after dinner or some yoga stretches before breakfast all add up and you will feel the benefits immediately.

The importance of strength training

Many of us midlifers are no strangers to long walks or yoga sessions – indeed, both are excellent forms of low-impact activity and should be part of our exercise armoury. The one area that's often neglected, however – let's face it, gyms can be intimidating – is strength training.

As we saw previously, countering age-related loss of muscle mass is critical to supporting your BMR. If you are exercising regularly but it doesn't seem to be as effective as it once was, then it would be a good idea to incorporate some strength training into your exercise regimen.

Another key benefit of strength training is that it protects against osteoporosis, a progressive condition characterised by increasingly fragile bones as we age. In later life, the rate at which our cells build new bone begins to slow down, leading to an overall loss of bone tissue. For women, the hormone oestrogen helps protect bone strength, so the decline of oestrogen in midlife also means a greater risk of osteoporosis.

Age UK reports that about 1 in 2 women and 1 in 5 men over 50 will break a bone because of osteoporosis, so it's important to keep our bones healthy.[40] According to a recent study that looked at the effects of resistance exercise on bone health, strength training was found to be the best strategy to improve muscle and bone mass in postmenopausal women, middle-aged men and the older population.[41]

Strength-training exercises work your muscles through resistance. This resistance can be provided by exercise equipment – such as weight machines at the gym, free weights/dumb-bells or resistance bands – or simply by using gravity and your own body weight.

Tips for planning exercise

Diarise: In the same way that it's important to plan your weekly meals, plan your exercise too. Sit down on a Sunday with your diary and figure out where you can slot your workouts in.

Be realistic: Don't try and do too much, otherwise you may become demotivated. It's far better to plan a few workouts that you actually do rather than a whole load that never happen.

Have fun: Another tip to stay on track with your exercise is to have fun. There's little point forcing yourself to do things you don't enjoy. Exercise can be a good way to socialise. So, find a tennis partner, go for a walk with a friend, meet someone for yoga and a coffee, or find a dog-walking pal.

Shake it up: Ideally, you will find a number of exercises you like, then you can mix them up. Pilates, yoga, high-intensity interval training (HIIT), tennis, walking, Zumba, CrossFit . . . there are so many choices these days, and lots of online options too.

Just do it: Nike was right about this: don't overthink it, pull on your gym gear and just do it. Procrastination is your enemy when it comes to exercise.

But don't overdo it: There are no medals on offer here! If you do too much exercise, you'll become exhausted and most likely injured. Rest is important – if you've had a big exercise session one day, keep it low-key the next. And the odd day off is good too!

Even if you don't have a gym membership, there are plenty of strength training workouts online that you can do at home with minimal equipment: a mat and a set of hand-weights are all you need. See the Resources section for some excellent free home workout websites and apps.

Pilates – the ultimate midlife exercise?

One form of exercise I am particularly fond of is Pilates and, judging by the packed classes I attend, it's not just me. I've had back problems since my late teens, which were worse after having children. A friend recommended doing Pilates (I can't remember who, but thank you!) and I quickly found that the benefits extended way beyond helping my back: I felt stronger, leaner and more flexible.

A good friend of mine, Roz, is a Pilates instructor and co-owner of Pilates & Co., a beautiful studio on the Gold Coast of Australia. Here, Roz explains why Pilates is so advantageous for us midlifers:

> Pilates is a great thing to include in your exercise programme as you get older because it is focused on strength, agility and flexibility – all of which can decrease as we age. Reformer Pilates is particularly beneficial because it incorporates resistance, which improves spine mobility, muscle mass and bone density.[42]

Roz also recommends mixing up Pilates with weight training and cardio, and making sure you have a rest day in between sessions to give your body time to recover. On your down days, you could go for a long walk or do some stretching or a light yoga session.

SLEEP

What happens to sleep quality as we age?

If there's one marker of the passing years, it's our changing sleep patterns. In our twenties we took sleep for granted; when our kids came along, we'd have sold a kidney for a decent lie-in; and now that our kids are finally sleeping in, we just can't seem to get a good night's kip.

Studies have shown that ageing is indeed associated with a decline in night-time sleep quality as well as with changes in the circadian regulation of the sleep-wake cycle.[43] What this means in plain English is that as we age, we find it harder to sleep, and when we do sleep, our quality of sleep is not as good as it once was.

Declining oestrogen levels in women can bring about night sweats and sleep apnoea, which disrupt sleep patterns and can lead to chronic sleep deprivation. In addition, our production of melatonin, the sleep hormone that regulates our sleep/wake cycle, also declines as we grow older, so it's no surprise that so many of us midlifers suffer from poor sleep.

The knock-on effects are not just detrimental to our mood; they aren't too good for our waistlines either. Increased daytime fatigue and low energy levels make it hard to make good food choices and inevitably lead to decreased physical activity. Unsurprisingly, in a study of more than 68,000 women over sixteen years, those who slept five hours or less per night gained more weight than those sleeping more than seven hours every night.[44]

What can we do to improve our quality of sleep?

Given the increased sleep challenges we face in midlife, it's worth taking a few steps to improve our 'sleep hygiene', as it's now known. There are a number of simple steps you can take, but possibly the biggest issue these days is our screens. Danielle North, author of *Pause: How to press pause before life does it for you*, advises:

> Stepping away from screens has positive benefits on improving the quality of our sleep. Screens, electrical devices and Wi-Fi emit artificial electromagnetic frequencies (EMF), which can disturb our natural sleep patterns. An easy habit to develop is to turn your smartphone off entirely (it still emits EMFs on airplane mode)

before you go to bed, and charge overnight in a different room and use the hub manager to set times when it turns off: 10pm to 8am, for example.[45]

Here are some other things you can try:

- **Keep to a routine.** Give yourself time to unwind before bed and aim for seven to eight hours of sleep each night. Even if you don't manage that, at least you've given yourself the best chance of a good night's sleep.
- **Exercise during the day** and in natural light. This will help regulate your circadian rhythm.
- **Keep your bedroom cool.** Rather than a duvet, have layers of bedcovers that you can adjust as necessary.
- **Invest in a comfortable pillow.** If you suffer neck discomfort, a comfortable, supportive gel or memory foam pillow can make a big difference.
- **Keep your bedroom dark.** If you don't have blackout blinds or curtains, think about getting some as you may be particularly light-sensitive.
- **Try a silk eye mask.** A comfortable silk eye mask can be a game-changer. Apparently, they can also help protect the delicate skin around the eyes and reduce fine lines. I can't vouch for that, but if they give you an extra hour or two of sleep, that's reason enough to invest.
- **Use ear plugs.** Once you've shut out the outside world, it's easier to power down your brain and drift off.
- **Aromatherapy.** Scent can be a sleep trigger, so try using a pillow spray or oil diffuser. Chamomile, lavender and vetiver are popular choices.
- **Sleep apps.** There are plenty of apps out there designed to help you sleep better – see the Resources section for some suggestions. By all means give them a go, but be aware that they might simply add another element of screen use before bed.

Can you eat your way to a better night's sleep?

According to the National Sleep Foundation, the difference between a restless and a restful night has a lot to do with the quality of our diet. It's important to provide our body with energy when it needs it most, so a nutritious breakfast will boost energy levels, but try not to eat a big meal too close to bedtime, as this will make it harder to drop off. Alcohol and caffeine are also best avoided later in the day.

Here are some other simple dietary adjustments that can help you to sleep better:

Melatonin, also known as the sleep hormone, lets your body know when it's time to sleep and when it's time to wake up. But as we grow older, melatonin levels decline. A few foods contain melatonin naturally – for example, milk, cherries, grapes, strawberries, tomatoes, peppers and pistachios – so these are all good things to eat in the evening.

Calcium and vitamin B6 are key micronutrients used in the production of melatonin. Calcium is found in high concentrations in dairy products, as well as leafy greens, so a glass of warm milk is a good choice of bedtime drink. Good sources of B6 include sunflower seeds, peanuts, oily fish, chicken, spinach and prunes.

Magnesium is another nutrient vital for sleep: not eating enough has been associated with higher levels of stress, anxiety and difficulty relaxing. Magnesium is found in almonds, leafy greens, bananas, avocado and fish.

And if all else fails . . .

- **Read a book.** This is still sound advice if you need to switch off before bed, but using an e-reader device could be part of the problem. Studies have shown that people using a light-emitting e-reader take longer to fall asleep, have reduced melatonin production, later timing of their circadian clock, and reduced alertness the next morning than when reading a printed book.[46]

STRESS

Stress can affect us at any stage of life, but the middle years usually bring their fair share of challenging life events. Many people in their forties and fifties can end up caught between the demands of looking after their own family as well as providing care to ageing relatives. For this reason they are often referred to as the 'sandwich generation'. This constant multitasking can be exhausting and leaves little time to focus on our own health and well-being.

Added to this, we are living and working longer: the retirement age for men and women in the UK is now 66 and many of us will need to keep working well beyond this to ensure a comfortable old age. It's likely that in midlife we will still be working long hours in demanding jobs. Midlife can be a stressful time, but how does it affect us from a health and weight management perspective, and what can we do about it?

What happens when we are stressed?

When we feel stressed, our nervous system instructs our body to release stress hormones, including adrenaline and cortisol, into our bloodstream. Apart from the short-term symptoms of extreme stress, such as quick, shallow breathing and increased heart rate and blood pressure, prolonged, elevated levels of stress hormones can have other deleterious effects on the body.

The cardiovascular system. If you experience stress over a long period of time, it can cause damage to blood vessels and arteries. This in turn elevates the risk of high blood pressure, heart attack and stroke.

The endocrine (hormone) system. Stress hormones trigger the production of blood sugar (glucose) to enable us to respond to stressful situations. This extra blood sugar is usually reabsorbed when the stress abates, but if stress is persistent there is an increased risk of diabetes in the longer term.

The gut. Stress is thought to cause a number of gut issues, including acid reflux, stomach pain, bloating, diarrhoea and constipation. Additionally, the gut's ability to absorb nutrients from our food may be reduced because of stress, which can lead to nutritional deficiencies.

The immune system. Cortisol released in our bodies suppresses the immune system and inflammatory pathways so we become more susceptible to infections and chronic inflammatory conditions.

The musculoskeletal system. Chronic stress causes our muscles to be in an almost constant state of tension. Prolonged muscle tension can cause aches and pains – and tense shoulders and neck may result in tension headaches and migraines.

The brain. Researchers believe that stress can cause inflammation in the brain, making the brain more susceptible to health problems such as Alzheimer's disease and other neurodegenerative conditions.[47]

Our emotional state. When we are stressed, we may feel more tired, have mood swings or feel more irritable than usual, and we may have difficulty falling or staying asleep.

How to recognise stress

According to the mental health charity Mind, the effects of stress can manifest in how we feel, how we behave and our physical health. Mind's website provides lots of information on the subject, including the following bullet lists to help you recognise the symptoms of stress.[48]

How you might feel:
- irritable, aggressive, impatient or wound up
- over-burdened
- anxious, nervous or afraid
- like your thoughts are racing and you can't switch off
- unable to enjoy yourself
- depressed
- uninterested in life
- like you've lost your sense of humour
- a sense of dread
- worried about your health
- neglected or lonely.

How you might be physically affected:
- shallow breathing or hyperventilating
- you might have a panic attack
- muscle tension
- blurred eyesight or sore eyes
- problems getting to sleep, staying asleep or having nightmares
- sexual problems, such as losing interest or being unable to enjoy sex
- tired all the time
- grinding your teeth or clenching your jaw
- headaches
- chest pain
- high blood pressure
- indigestion or heartburn
- constipation or diarrhoea
- feeling sick, dizzy or fainting.

How might you behave? You might:

- find it hard to make decisions
- worry constantly
- avoid situations that are troubling you
- snap at people
- bite your nails
- pick at your skin
- be unable to concentrate
- eat too much or too little
- smoke or drink alcohol more than usual
- feel restless, as if you can't sit still
- be tearful or cry a lot.

The techniques for stress reduction outlined below are useful for mild stress relief, but if you are experiencing any of the above symptoms it would be sensible to seek advice from your GP.

How can we reduce midlife stress?

While there may not be much we can do about the causes of our stress – we have to keep caring for our family and earning a living, after all – we can control how we respond to stressors. Here are some daily practices that may help.

Prioritise. No matter how busy we are, it's not worth sacrificing our health and happiness. Learn to say no to things that aren't essential. If you don't reply to every email in your inbox each day, so be it. At home, delegate tasks and get your family to help out more. Reset your own expectations and the expectations of those around you.

Stay positive. One of the things we have going for us in midlife, thanks to our life experience, is perspective. One phrase I use a lot is that nothing is ever as good or as bad as it first appears – or, as my grandmother would say, everything comes out in the wash!

Meditate. Meditation comes in many guises. It can be sitting cross-legged and chanting, as per the cliché, but it can equally be a few moments of quiet contemplation (there are some good meditation apps available), listening to some uplifting music or relaxing in a warm bath. See meditation as a mental 'time out' from the stresses of everyday life, which brings mental as well as physical benefits.

Exercise. Exercise is absolutely the best thing for stress-busting: it boosts oxygen circulation and the production of 'feel good' endorphins. Even if you don't have masses of energy, simply taking a walk outside, preferably in nature, has been shown to reduce cortisol levels.[49]

Eat well. Of course! See the box below for suggestions.

Can what we eat help to reduce stress?

Foods can help reduce stress in a number of ways. Some boost serotonin levels (this is also known as the 'happy hormone'). Others reduce levels of the stress hormones cortisol and adrenaline. Here are some of my favourites:

- **Eggs** contain the essential amino acid tryptophan which can help the body to produce more serotonin.
- **Avocados** are rich in stress-relieving B vitamins and heart-healthy fats, which may help to lessen anxiety.
- **Almonds** contain vitamins B2 and E, which help support the immune system in times of stress.
- **Oranges** contain lots of vitamin C, which helps to lower blood pressure and reduce cortisol levels.
- **Spinach** is rich in magnesium. Not eating enough magnesium can trigger headaches and fatigue, compounding the effects of stress.
- **Dark chocolate** (over 70% cocoa solids). Cocoa polyphenols have been shown to reduce stress, especially in women.[50] Hurrah!

ALCOHOL

A drop of red wine is good for you, isn't it? Surely all those French octogenarians can't be wrong! Or can they? The idea that red wine is a factor in longevity stems from observational studies of the 'French paradox', a term used to describe the relatively low incidence of cardiovascular disease in the French population, despite a relatively high-fat diet.

More recent studies have found that the benefits are not confined to red wine, and that a moderate consumption of any type of alcohol lowers your risk of developing heart disease and Type 2 diabetes.[51] It has even been shown to help prevent gallstones.[52]

Alcohol and the menopause

But what about when we hit the menopause? Do alcohol and the menopause mix, or are they a cocktail best avoided? The North American Menopause Society advises that midlife women who drink moderately have a lower risk of Type 2 diabetes, dementia and stroke and have stronger bones than non-drinkers[53] – for older women at risk of osteoporosis, this is good to know.

The heart benefits of moderate drinking become apparent around the menopause (when the risk of heart disease in women increases) and continue afterwards. Interestingly, these protective benefits still apply if you are on HRT. But for many women any potential heart health benefits have to be balanced against a small increased risk of breast cancer for those who drink even the smallest quantity of alcohol.

To put this in perspective, a woman in later life is ten times more likely to die from heart disease than from breast cancer so the heart benefits may outweigh the small increased cancer risk. However, for anyone who's at higher risk of breast cancer (women with a family history of genetic breast cancers, etc.), it may be better to avoid alcohol altogether.

Drink smart

White wine. Choose lower (12% or less) Alcohol By Volume (ABV) wines, such as sparkling or dry white wines. Diluting wine by adding sparkling water to make a spritzer is a smart way to slash calories, lower alcohol levels, and stay hydrated.

Red wine. Red wine has all the lovely health-giving poly-phenols but generally has a higher ABV, so keep an eye on the units. Opt for a lighter style like Pinot Noir.

Clear spirits with mixers. Gin or vodka with low-calorie mixers are another good option. There are some excellent mixers on the market these days that aren't packed with artificial sweeteners and chemicals.

Low ABV Kombucha. Kombucha is a fermented drink which is often alcohol-free but there are some that are naturally low in alcohol (1–2% ABV). It's also good for the gut!

Cocktails. You can still enjoy a cocktail, but try adding less alcohol and lose the sugar:

- **Not So Bloody Mary:** If you keep the vodka content low and the veggie level high, you can still enjoy this classic cocktail.
- **Low-Cal Cosmo:** 1 shot of vodka, soda water and a splash of lime and cranberry juice.
- **Moscow Mule Light:** 1 shot vodka, light ginger beer, lime juice and lots of ice.
- **Low Mo:** For a healthier mojito, mix 1 shot white rum with lime juice, soda water and fresh mint leaves. Use stevia drops – a plant-based sweetener with zero calories – instead of sugar for sweetness.

It's worth noting that, whereas light to moderate drinking does seem to convey some health benefits, heavy drinking does the reverse. The risk of heart disease, cancer, Type 2 diabetes, dementia and stroke increases if you drink more than the recommended limits – in fact, heavy drinking can lead to irreversible osteoporosis.

Drinking may also trigger hot flushes, but the evidence for this is inconsistent – some studies have shown that alcohol actually decreases night sweats – so you need to determine whether alcohol is a trigger for you personally or not.

Men and midlife drinking

A recent review of qualitative research into midlife male drinking found that in England and Scotland middle-aged men are the demographic with the highest average weekly alcohol consumption, and men are disproportionately negatively affected by alcohol.[54] The latest figures show that in the UK rates of alcohol-specific deaths in men are more than double those in women.[55]

The motivators identified for drinking among this cohort include relaxation, socialising and maintenance of male friendships. Midlife men tend to see their drinking as social and a choice, in contrast to 'problem drinkers', whose alcohol consumption negatively impacts their lives and the people around them.

Unfortunately, heavier drinking increases the risk of developing some cancers, heart disease, high blood pressure, cirrhosis of the liver and alcohol dependence. A report in the journal *Neurology* also found a link between heavy drinking and cognitive decline: compared with men who didn't drink or who drank moderately, mental decline began to appear one to six years earlier in men who averaged more than 2.5 drinks a day.[56]

How much is too much?

For both men and women, any potential health benefits are only associated with low to moderate drinking. Current UK government advice is to stick to a maximum of 14 units a week and have no more than 6 units in one session. More than this is considered a 'binge', and the health risks increase significantly. Finally, have at least three drink-free days a week, ideally two consecutively.

If you aren't sure how much you're drinking, you could download a tracking app on your phone. You might be surprised by how quickly the units add up. Here's the alcohol content of some popular drinks:

- gin and tonic (25ml measure) – 1 unit
- 120ml glass of champagne or sparkling wine – 1.5 units
- 150ml glass of 12% ABV white wine – 1.8 units
- 150ml glass of 14% ABV red wine – 2.1 units
- a pint of 4% beer – 2.3 units.

Deciding whether or not to drink, especially for 'medicinal purposes', requires careful consideration of the health benefits and risks. We each have a unique set of risk factors so it's important to take these into account when considering our alcohol consumption.

What about alcohol and weight loss?

Alcohol is notoriously calorific and is often a dieter's downfall. Because it's in liquid form, it's far too easy to quaff enough calories to sabotage our weight-loss efforts without realising it. Some people feel that calories in drinks somehow 'don't count' or aren't 'equal' to those that we eat. So does the body metabolise drinks any differently from food, or is that just a case of wishful thinking?

The science around how our bodies digest alcohol is complicated. Some studies suggest that the calories in alcohol may not be entirely available to the body because alcohol is treated as a toxin and so at a certain point the alcohol is excreted rather than digested.

However, because calories taken in liquid form aren't as filling, the calories we drink can rack up at an alarming rate if we don't keep an eye on them: a large glass of wine (250ml) with 13% ABV can add 228 calories to our dinner.[57]

With this in mind, it's worth seeking out lower-calorie drinks and avoiding those that pack a particularly heavy calorific punch (see p. 67). Sweet or creamy cocktails, alcopops, dessert wine and liqueurs are all best avoided while you're trying to lose weight.

The other problem with drinking too much is that it increases hunger and appetite – late night cheese-on-toast frenzies don't help our waistlines, and having a hangover doesn't generally lead to good food choices or an inclination to exercise.

The bottom line is, if you are trying to lose weight you don't have to give up alcohol completely. As long as you keep an eye on the calories, you can still enjoy a tipple or two. Just be sure to choose your drink with care and don't give in to the late-night munchies.

The Recipes

And now for my favourite part of the book: the food!

Many people make the mistake of confusing 'healthy' food with 'diet' food – boring salads, minuscule portions or unappetising low-fat versions of things that leave you hungry and craving all the foods you've been told to avoid. This is clearly unsustainable, and that's why the secret to healthy eating, and ultimately to losing weight, lies in discovering healthy whole foods that you love. The converse is also true: just because something is healthy, it doesn't follow that you *have* to eat it. There's a huge choice of delicious, nutritious food out there, so seek out the ones you really enjoy eating. Don't like porridge? Fine – maybe granola is more your thing. Not a kale fan? Me neither; I prefer spinach.

It has been my mission with *The Midlife Method* to create easy, crowd-pleasing recipes that are naturally low-calorie and macro-balanced – but, more importantly, also delicious. I have spoken to many fellow midlifers who desperately want to get to grips with their diet and drop a few pounds but have found it hard to balance feeding their family with their own weight-loss goals.

Don't let this be an obstacle. Generally speaking, breakfast and lunch aren't too difficult to navigate: porridge, avocado on toast, a healthy soup or salad are all easy to prepare. Where things can come unstuck is dinner-time, so most of the meal recipes I've devised are family-friendly, with swaps, Tips & Tweaks and additions so you can accommodate your family's likes and dislikes.

For the next few weeks, food needs to take centre stage. But, as you get used to the recipes, swapping between Light Days and Regular Days and finding your favourite meal combinations, it will get easier, eventually becoming second nature.

There is one important new habit you will need to develop, if you don't do it already, and that is meal planning.

MEAL PLANNING

Doing a meal plan every weekend and making a list for your weekly shop or online order is without doubt one of the foundations of eating well. Without it, things can quickly veer off-track and you may end up resorting to convenience foods or calorie-laden takeaways. With a small amount of effort and prep at the weekend, you can eat well all week.

You can either combine the recipes in this book to create your own meal plans *or* use the Light Day Meal Combos (p. 250) and Regular Day Meal Combos (p. 254) to form the basis of your meal plan. Or, for ultimate ease, you can follow the Four-Week Meal Plan (p. 258), which includes the optimal combination of Light and Regular Days.

To recap:

- ✓ Light Days – 800 calories
- ✓ Regular Days – 1,600 calories (woman)/2,000 (man)
- ✓ Week 1 – six Light Days/one Regular Day
- ✓ Week 2 – five Light Days/two Regular Days
- ✓ Week 3 – four Light Days/three Regular Days
- ✓ Week 4 – three Light Days/four Regular Days.

Meal prep – how to get ahead

You've done your meal plan, now have a look at the recipes you've chosen and see if there's anything you can make in advance to get a jump-start on the week:

Make soup, curry or a stew in advance. Make plenty of it, keep some in the fridge and freeze the rest – that's a load of quick meals sorted. Try the Carrot, Lemon & Ginger Soup (p. 146) or the Quickest Ever Spinach & Chickpea Curry (p. 206).

Make a dip/spread. It only takes about ten minutes to make a dip or spread, and they are handy for a quick lunch or healthy snack (with cut-up veggies). Try the Coronation Hummus (p. 126), which is also excellent in a wrap.

Roast some veg. This is virtually effortless: with a stash in the fridge, you have the wherewithal for a delicious and nutritious salad or side dish at a moment's notice. Try the Paprika Roast Cauli & Sweet Potatoes with Feta (p. 200).

Boil some eggs. A quick egg sandwich or a hard-boiled egg peeled and quartered on a salad are lunchtime lifesavers.

Make some Spicy Seeds Topper. These are brilliant for pimping any savoury dish – things on toast, soup, salads, on eggs, etc. (p. 122).

Make some granola. I cannot tell you what a game-changer homemade granola is. My Go-to Granola (p. 89) is nutty, crunchy and completely sugar-free.

KITCHEN TIPS

No matter how experienced you are in the kitchen, it's easy to fall into lazy habits. I know I do! These simple tips will make life much easier when it's time to cook:

1. Read the recipe right through before you begin, including the Tips & Tweaks section. It seems obvious, but how often do we plough straight in and then realise something needs to be defrosted or cooked in advance, or we haven't allowed enough time for marinating?

2. Get out all the equipment you're going to need before you begin – bowls, pans, knives, a chopping board, a grater, the food processor/blender/mixer, scales, measuring cups or spoons. You don't want to be digging around in cupboards and drawers with your hands covered in food.

3. Get out all the ingredients you're going to need before you start cooking. It's annoying to get halfway through a recipe and realise you are missing a key ingredient or have something burning on the hob as you ferret around at the back of the fridge for the next ingredient.

4. Preheat the oven, if required, boil the kettle for stock or put a pan of water on if you need one. Also make sure any baking dishes, tins or trays are out and prepared if they need to be greased or lined.

5. Have a container on the kitchen worktop to put the detritus in as you go. Have a clean cloth for wiping down and a tea towel at the ready.

NOTES ON THE RECIPES

Calories per serving and macro breakdown

At the top of each recipe, the calorie count is given (per serving). This will help you plan your meals for the day (800 calories on a Light Day, 1,600 (woman)/2,000 (man) on a Regular Day). Also listed is the percentage macro breakdown. You don't need to pay too much attention to this – if you're using recipes from this book, the macros will average out over the course of the week to roughly 30% fat, 25% protein and 45% carbs.

Prep time and cooking time

None of the recipes are particularly involved or time-consuming, but it's helpful to have a rough idea of how long a particular dish will take to prepare. We all work at different speeds, so the prep times are generous.

Quantity/serves

It's important to pay attention to portion sizes to ensure you are hitting your calorie allowances. This may require you to weigh your food, but generally you can divide up meals by eye. Obviously, if a recipe serves two then one serving will be half what the recipe makes.

Dietary restrictions

Where recipes are vegan, vegetarian, dairy-free or gluten-free, this is indicated, but if you are already following a restricted diet I would advise consulting your GP or a dietitian before embarking on a weight-loss programme, to ensure your nutritional requirements are being met.

Ingredients and method

Brown sugar: Unless otherwise specified, 'brown sugar' refers to light or dark brown sugar, so use what you have.

Butter: In recipes where butter is given as an ingredient, this means regular salted butter unless otherwise stated.

Greek yogurt: Where the recipe states 'Greek yogurt', this refers to 0% fat, plain, unsweetened Greek yogurt. This is to minimise calories on Light Days. On Regular Days you can use a higher fat percentage Greek yogurt if you prefer it.

Olive oil: If a recipe simply states 'olive oil', this means the regular 'light' style of olive oil that you can use for cooking. If extra virgin olive oil is required, it will be specified in the recipe.

Neutral oil: Where the recipe refers to 'neutral oil' this means a flavourless oil that can be used for cooking at a high heat. I like to use organic rapeseed oil as it is one of the healthiest.

Stock: Where stock is listed, this is stock made from stock cubes (assume that one cube makes 500ml of stock). Of course, you can substitute fresh stock if you wish. I have assumed in the calorie counts that 500ml stock adds around 35 calories to the dish. Fresh stocks may add more.

Seasoning: The recipes are created to my taste in terms of the addition of salt and pepper. All seasoning can be adjusted to your preference – and you may even wish to leave salt out if you're trying to reduce sodium in your diet for health reasons.

Oven temperatures: All oven temperatures are given in degrees centigrade (°C) for a fan-assisted oven. Please adjust as necessary for your oven.

Tips & Tweaks

The Tips & Tweaks section of each recipe gives preparation tips, serving suggestions, and other ideas for how to adapt the recipe for Light and Regular Days and to make it suitable for other family members. Be sure to read this section before you start cooking.

Where I suggest side dishes or additions to the recipes, you can find the relevant calorie counts in the 'Calorie-counted sides and additions' charts on pp. 287–90.

RECIPE LISTING

Breakfast & brunch

The Recipes

Meals by calorie count

The Recipes

Sweet stuff & snacks

BREAKFAST & BRUNCH

Rhubarb, Apple & Ginger Compote

I think it's a peculiarly midlife thing to love ginger. As a kid, I remember seeing the adults eating crystallised stem ginger from a jar and thinking it was such a bizarre thing to eat, but something happens to those taste buds as we age, and now I can't get enough of the stuff. It's an excellent companion to rhubarb, and I've added apple for sweetness and texture.

Quantity/serves: 10 × 50g (2 tbsp) servings

Calories per serving: 30

Prep time: 10 mins

Cooking time: 30 mins

☑ Vegan   ☑ Lacto-Ovo Vegetarian

☑ Dairy-Free   ☑ Gluten-Free

Fat 4%
Protein 4%
Carbs 92%

Ingredients

250g rhubarb, trimmed and chopped
250g apples, peeled, cored and chopped
1 tsp vanilla extract
3cm piece of fresh root ginger, peeled and finely grated
¼ tsp cinnamon, or 1 cinnamon stick broken in two
2 star anise (optional)
2 tbsp maple syrup or sweetener of choice (optional)

Method

Place all the ingredients, except the maple syrup, in a large saucepan, along with 1 tablespoon water. Cover loosely with a lid and simmer over a low heat for 20–30 minutes, until the rhubarb and apple have broken down – you will need to stir occasionally, and perhaps add a drop more water if it's getting too dry or sticking. Leave to cool slightly, then remove the cinnamon stick (if using) and star anise. Add the maple syrup or sweetener to taste and mix well. This will keep for up to 2 weeks in the fridge.

Tips & Tweaks

- Make this at the weekend and keep it in the fridge to pep up your breakfasts all week long.
- Can be eaten warm or kept in the fridge and eaten cold, or reheated.
- My favourite way to eat this is stirred into Greek yogurt with a sprinkling of My Go-to Granola (p. 89) over the top (approx. 225 cals).

Quick Berry Sauce

This is one of those simple recipes that, once you've made it, becomes a breakfast mainstay. It's delicious over yogurt, on pancakes or stirred into porridge. And needless to say, it's full of health-boosting berry goodness.

Quantity/serves: 4

Calories per serving: 39

Prep time: **3 mins**

Cooking time: **7 mins**

☑ Vegan   ☑ Lacto-Ovo Vegetarian

☑ Dairy-Free   ☑ Gluten-Free

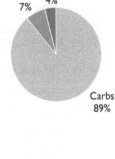

Fat 7%   Protein 4%   Carbs 89%

Ingredients

200g frozen mixed berries
1 tbsp maple syrup

Method

Place all the ingredients in a medium-sized saucepan and add 1 tablespoon water. Place over a low heat and simmer for around 5 minutes until the fruit has defrosted and heated through. Mash lightly with a fork, and add a little more water if necessary, to loosen.

Tips & Tweaks

- This sauce is delicious served straight away while warm, but you can keep it in the fridge for a few days and eat it cold. It's particularly nice with yogurt this way.

The Healthiest Pancakes in the World

I've been making simple pancakes with oats, banana and eggs for the longest time. One day, I saw a picture of some beautiful green pancakes and it inspired me to throw in a handful of baby spinach. The spinach doesn't affect the taste or texture; it just adds gorgeous green nutrition.

Quantity/serves: 2

Calories per serving: 160

Prep time: **5 mins**

Cooking time: **12 mins**

☒ Vegan ☑ Lacto-Ovo Vegetarian

☑ Dairy-Free ☑ Gluten-Free (use GF oats)

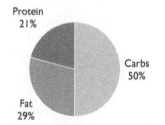

Ingredients

> 1 large or 2 small ripe bananas, peeled
> 2 eggs
> a handful of baby spinach leaves (approx. 50g)
> 2 tbsp rolled oats
> a drop of neutral oil or spray oil (if needed)

Method

Put the banana(s), eggs, spinach and oats in a blender and blend for about 1 minute until the mixture is really smooth and of a pourable consistency. Add a little water to loosen if required.

Heat a large non-stick pan over a medium heat. If it's a good pan, you won't need any cooking oil, but if you do, just add a drop of oil to the pan (or give it a light spray if you have a spray oil). Once the pan is hot, pour palm-sized amounts of batter into the pan – or you can make thinner, crêpe-style pancakes if your batter is thinner.

Cook for a minute or two until golden, then flip over and cook for a minute or so on the other side, then remove from the pan and set aside while you make the next pancake. Continue until you have used up all the batter.

Tips & Tweaks

- This is a great way to use up sweet, overripe bananas.
- These are wonderful served with Quick Berry Sauce (p. 86; 39 cals per serving) or some fresh strawberries and blueberries.

My Go-to Granola

Cast your mind back to a time before granola, where a healthy breakfast was a bowl of Special K! How times have changed. Granola has been brightening up our breakfast bowls for some time now, but the problem is that some of them contain a lot of sugar. This one doesn't, but it still delivers exceptional crunch. A word to the wise: it's calorific, so go easy.

Quantity/serves: 10 × 40g servings

Calories per serving: 165

Prep time: **10 mins**

Cooking time: **40 mins**

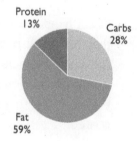

Protein 13%
Carbs 28%
Fat 59%

☒ Vegan   ☑ Lacto-Ovo Vegetarian

☑ Dairy-Free   ☑ Gluten-Free (use GF oats)

Ingredients

Plain
3 egg whites
100g jumbo oats
50g raw, unsalted cashew nuts, chopped
50g Brazil nuts, chopped
50g flaked almonds
25g flax seeds
25g sunflower or pumpkin seeds
a pinch of salt

Variations

- **Cinnamon & Coconut:** Add 1 tsp ground cinnamon and 3 tbsp unsweetened coconut flakes or desiccated coconut.
- **Orange & Ginger:** Add the finely grated zest of ½ orange and 1 tsp ground ginger.

Method

Preheat the oven to 150°C/gas mark 2 and line a baking tray with baking parchment.

Use a hand mixer or a stand mixer to whisk the egg whites until they form stiff peaks. In a separate bowl, mix together all the remaining ingredients, including any extra ingredients for the variations. Add the whisked egg whites to this mixture and stir thoroughly with a metal spoon to ensure everything is evenly coated.

Spread out the mixture in an even layer on the prepared baking tray and bake for 40 minutes, stirring after 20 minutes to break up the granola a little. Leave to cool fully, then store in an airtight container. It will keep for up to 3 weeks.

Tips & Tweaks

- The classic way to eat granola is with yogurt and fruit (add one serving of granola to 2 tbsp Greek yogurt and add a handful of berries – approx. 225 calories in total), or with a serving of Rhubarb, Apple & Ginger Compote (p. 84; 1 serving = 30 cals).
- This also makes a nice dessert on a Regular Day, served with oven-roasted stone fruits.

Indian Spiced Omelette Wrap

I am on a constant mission to find new ways to eat eggs. Once I realised they were the key to powering me through my mid-morning munchies, they have become an almost daily ritual. It's hard to believe that not so long ago, we were being advised to eat just one egg a week! Happily, those days are long gone, and current advice is that you can eat as many eggs as you like. I honestly don't think you'll find a better way to eat them than this, so let's get cracking!

Quantity/serves: 2

Calories per serving: 167

Prep time: 10 mins

Cooking time: 5 mins

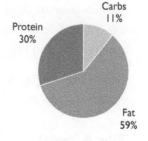

Protein 30%
Carbs 11%
Fat 59%

☒ Vegan   ☑ Lacto-Ovo Vegetarian

☑ Dairy-Free   ☑ Gluten-Free

Ingredients

4 eggs
½ tsp ground cumin
½ tsp ground turmeric
1 tsp neutral oil
½ small red pepper, diced
2 spring onions, sliced
1 small tomato, diced
a pinch of salt
a pinch of freshly ground black pepper

Method

Break the eggs into a bowl and whisk them lightly with a fork. Add the cumin and turmeric and whisk again to combine.

Place a large, non-stick pan over a medium heat and add the oil. Add the red pepper and sauté for 1–2 minutes, just to soften, then add the spring onions and tomato and cook for a further minute. Remove the mixture from the pan and set aside in a bowl.

Return the pan to the heat. Give the egg mixture another good stir and pour half of it over the base of the pan. Season well with salt and pepper. Cook for 1–2 minutes, then loosen with a spatula and flip over to cook lightly on the other side for 30 seconds. Place the cooked omelette on a plate. Give the remaining egg mixture another stir and repeat to make a second omelette.

Divide the veggie mixture between the two omelettes, roll each one up like a wrap and cut in half to serve.

Tips & Tweaks

- Save time in the morning by chopping up the veggies and whisking up the eggs with the spices the night before, then store in airtight containers in the fridge until you're ready to cook.
- Serve with some Greek yogurt (1 tbsp = 15 cals) and a few dried chilli flakes.

Oaty Miracle Muffins

If you are a porridge lover, these oaty little muffins are sure to be a big breakfast hit. I've given three ideas for flavour combinations below, but the options are endless. Just mix up your favourite combo (you can even do this the night before) and, with just a couple of minutes in the microwave in the morning, brekkie is ready.

Quantity/serves: makes 2 muffins

Calories per serving: 167

Prep time: 5 mins

Cooking time: 2–3 mins (microwave) or 20–25 mins (oven)

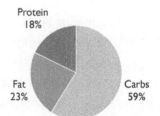

☒ Vegan   ☑ Lacto-Ovo Vegetarian

☑ Dairy-Free   ☑ Gluten-Free (use GF oats)

Ingredients

Berry & Cinnamon
1 ripe banana
1 egg
30g rolled oats
100ml semi-skimmed milk
½ tsp ground cinnamon
50g fresh blueberries or raspberries

Variations

Instead of cinnamon and berries:

- **Dark Chocolate & Peanut Butter (254 cals per muffin):** Mash 1 tbsp peanut butter in with the egg and banana, then stir in 20g dark chocolate chips instead of the berries.
- **Carrot & Raisin (182 cals per muffin):** Stir in 1 tbsp finely grated carrot and 20g raisins instead of the berries.

Method

In a mixing bowl, mash together the banana and egg. Add the oats, milk and cinnamon and combine well to form a batter. Gently stir in the fruit. Divide the batter between two silicone muffin cases, ramekins, mugs or other microwave-proof containers. Microwave on high for 2 minutes, then check that they are fully cooked. If needed, give them another 30 seconds or so (the exact cooking time will depend on the container you use and your microwave).

Alternatively, to bake them in the oven, divide the batter between two silicone muffin cases or other ovenproof containers. Preheat the oven to 180°C/gas mark 4 and bake for 20–25 minutes.

Remove the muffins from their containers or cases and eat straight away.

Tips & Tweaks

- Mix up the batter the night before for super speedy results in the morning.
- For extra sweetness, drizzle over some date syrup, maple syrup or honey (for each, 1 tsp = 17 cals).
- If you like a tangier topping, try a dollop of Greek yogurt (1 tbsp = 15 cals).

Apple & Carrot Basic Bircher

Overnight oats have become a thing of late, but it all started with the original Swiss Bircher muesli. This is a fairly traditional rendition, but I've added finely grated carrot for extra flavour, sweetness and nutrition. This is my fallback breakfast because you can make a load on a Sunday night and eat it over the course of the week.

Quantity/serves: 3

Calories per serving: 182

Prep time: 10–15 mins

Cooking time: 0 mins

☒ Vegan   ☑ Lacto-Ovo Vegetarian

☒ Dairy-Free   ☑ Gluten-Free (use GF oats)

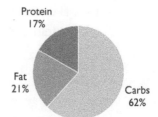

Protein 17%

Fat 21%

Carbs 62%

Ingredients

½ red apple, skin on, grated (use large grater)
1 small carrot, peeled and grated (use fine grater)
75g rolled oats
250ml semi-skimmed milk (or your milk of choice)
15g raisins
¼ tsp ground cinnamon
2 heaped tsp mixed raw seeds (such as flax,
    sunflower, pumpkin or sesame)
a pinch of salt

Method

Simply place all the ingredients in an airtight container with a lid. Mix well, cover with the lid and pop in the fridge overnight. This will keep for several days.

Tips & Tweaks

- This is the perfect Light Day breakfast as it's really filling and nutritious.
- I like to stir in 1 tablespoon Greek yogurt, which adds more protein and calcium (1 tbsp = 15 cals).

Brilliant Breakfast Muffins

Cake for breakfast? Yes please! But this isn't any old cake: the butter and sugar have been reduced and the fibre upped to make this a delicious but lower-GI option, meaning that it won't spike your blood sugar like regular muffins will. And even better, the calorie count sneaks in at just under 200.

Quantity/serves: 8 muffins

Calories per serving: 193

Prep time: 10 mins

Cooking time: 20–25 mins

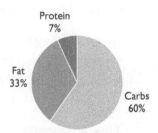

☒ Vegan   ☑ Lacto-Ovo Vegetarian

☒ Dairy-Free   ☒ Gluten-Free

Ingredients

    40g butter
    100g brown sugar
    1 large egg
    100ml semi-skimmed milk
    50g plain wholemeal flour
    50g plain flour
    25g rolled oats
    25g unsweetened, desiccated coconut
    2 tsp baking powder
    1 tsp mixed spice or ground cinnamon (optional)
    150g (approx. 2 small) bananas, peeled and lightly
        mashed

Method

Preheat the oven to 180°C/gas mark 4 and place 8 muffin cases in a muffin tin.

Using a hand mixer or stand mixer, cream together the butter and sugar, then add the egg and milk and combine well. Add the wholemeal and plain flour, along with the oats, coconut, baking powder and mixed spice or cinnamon (if using) and mix together on a low speed to make sure everything is incorporated. Now add the mashed bananas and stir in well with a metal spoon.

Spoon the batter equally into the muffin cases and bake for 20–25 minutes until golden brown on top and firm to the touch. These can be eaten warm or left to cool.

Tips & Tweaks

- These freeze well in an airtight container; just remove from the freezer 1 hour before eating.
- Have one for breakfast on a Light Day, or as a healthy snack on a Regular Day.
- These are lovely paired with some chopped fresh fruit or berries.

Baked Bacon & Eggs with Asparagus Dippers

When I created this recipe, I actually drew a smiley face on my recipe testing sheet. So simple, so delicious and about as far away from 'diet food' as you could possibly get. This is my new Saturday go-to breakfast.

Quantity/serves: 2

Calories per serving: 194

Prep time: 10 mins

Cooking time: 15 mins

☒ Vegan   ☒ Lacto-Ovo Vegetarian

☑ Dairy-Free   ☑ Gluten-Free

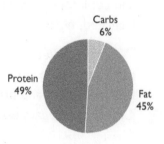

Carbs 6%

Protein 49%

Fat 45%

Ingredients

drop of olive oil, for greasing
4 back bacon rashers, any excess fat trimmed
4 eggs
a pinch of salt
a pinch of freshly ground black pepper
8 asparagus spears, woody ends trimmed

Method

Preheat the oven to 180°C/gas mark 4 and lightly grease 4 holes of a muffin tin with a drop of olive oil.

Place a frying pan over a high heat and add the bacon. Fry for 1 minute on each side until just cooked through, then transfer the rashers to a plate lined with kitchen roll to soak up any excess grease.

Use the bacon rashers to line the greased muffin tin holes (you can tear the rashers if needed). Break an egg into each one and sprinkle with salt and pepper, then place in the oven. Check after 10 minutes: the white should be cooked, but the yolks still runny. Cook for a few more minutes if necessary.

Meanwhile, half-fill a small saucepan with water and place over a medium heat. Bring to the boil, then add the asparagus spears and cook for 1–2 minutes, just to soften: you want them lightly blanched, not soggy.

When the baked eggs are done, remove from the oven and gently run a knife around the edges of the muffin holes to loosen. Lift out the baked eggs and place on serving plates. Serve 2 per person, with 4 asparagus spears each as dippers.

Tips & Tweaks

- Sprinkle over some dried chilli flakes for extra pizzazz.
- On a Regular Day, add a nice slice of sourdough (1 slice = 100 cals).

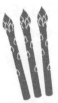

Chorizo Omelette

Chorizo and eggs are a fabulous combination. Just add some spring onion, red pepper and cherry tomatoes, and you have an omelette fit for a king (well a king on a Light Day, at least!). Pair with a slice of sourdough for a leisurely Regular Day brunch.

Quantity/serves: 2

Calories per serving: 208

Prep time: 5 mins

Cooking time: 7 mins

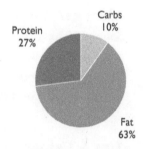

Protein 27%
Carbs 10%
Fat 63%

☒ Vegan   ☒ Lacto-Ovo Vegetarian

☑ Dairy-Free   ☑ Gluten-Free

Ingredients

2 large eggs
50g chorizo, skin removed, roughly chopped
1 spring onion, finely sliced
½ red pepper, finely sliced
10 cherry tomatoes, halved
a pinch of salt
a pinch of freshly ground black pepper

Method

Crack the eggs into a jug, add a splash of water and whisk together with a fork.

Place the chorizo in a medium-sized, non-stick frying pan over a low heat and cook for around 1 minute, until the fat starts to release. Add the spring onion, red pepper and cherry tomatoes and continue to fry gently for a few minutes until softened.

Add the whisked eggs and season with salt and pepper. Cook for a couple of minutes until the omelette is golden underneath, then flip and give the other side a few seconds, just to set any still-raw egg. Remove the omelette from the pan and divide into two. Place each half on a plate and serve.

Tips & Tweaks

- Sprinkle over some Spicy Seeds Topper (p. 122; 1 tsp = 20 cals) for extra crunchy heat.
- This is perfect as is for a Light Day breakfast. On a Regular Day, add a slice of sourdough or seedy toast (1 slice = 100 cals).

Big Mushrooms

Those enormous portobello mushrooms can be intimidating, but roasting them is so easy, and the intense, earthy flavour they develop is amazing. This recipe lends itself to breakfast but honestly, I'd eat it any time of the day.

Quantity/serves: 2

Calories per serving: 210

Prep time: 5 mins

Cooking time: 20 mins

☒ Vegan ☑ Lacto-Ovo Vegetarian

☑ Dairy-Free ☑ Gluten-Free

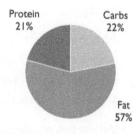

Protein 21%
Carbs 22%
Fat 57%

Ingredients

2 large portobello mushrooms
1 tsp olive oil
2 thick slices from a large (beef) tomato
150g spinach leaves
2 eggs, whisked
a pinch of salt
a pinch of freshly ground black pepper
½ avocado, peeled, stoned and sliced

Method

Preheat the oven to 200°C/gas mark 6.

Rub the mushrooms with the olive oil and place on a baking sheet, stem side up. Gently lay a slice of tomato on each mushroom and place in the oven to roast for 20 minutes.

Meanwhile, place a frying pan over a low heat and add the spinach leaves. Wilt gently, then turn off the heat until you're ready to cook the eggs.

About 5 minutes before the mushrooms will be ready, place the pan over a medium heat, with the spinach still in it. Add the whisked eggs and season well with salt and pepper. Fold gently with a spatula a few times to scramble.

When the mushrooms are done, remove them from the oven and place each one on a plate. Top with the spinach and scrambled egg mixture, arrange the avocado slices on the side and serve.

Tips & Tweaks

- Sprinkle over some Spicy Seeds Topper (p. 122; 1 tsp = 20 cals) for extra flavour and texture.
- Add a slice of sourdough for a super weekend Regular Day brunch (1 slice = 100 cals).

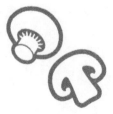

Spinachy Baked Eggs

You've seen shakshuka all over the place, I'm sure, and it's one of my favourite weekend breakfast recipes, so I had to include it in this book. This version packs all the flavour of the original with the minimum number of ingredients. The only addition (for added nutrition) is the spinach.

Quantity/serves: 2

Calories per serving: 242

Prep time: 10 mins

Cooking time: 30 mins

☒ Vegan   ☑ Lacto-Ovo Vegetarian

☑ Dairy-Free   ☑ Gluten-Free

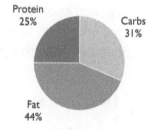

Protein 25%
Carbs 31%
Fat 44%

Ingredients

1 tsp olive oil
1 small red onion, finely sliced
1 garlic clove, crushed
1 large red pepper, chopped
400g can chopped tomatoes
½ tsp dried chilli flakes (or more, to taste)
½ tsp ground cumin
½ tsp paprika
½ tsp brown sugar
a squeeze of lemon juice
100g baby spinach leaves
4 eggs
a good pinch of salt
a good pinch of freshly ground black pepper

Method

Place a medium-sized frying pan over a low heat and add the oil. Add the onion and sauté for a few minutes until it begins to soften. Add the garlic and continue to sauté, then add the red pepper and cook for 5 minutes until softened. Stir in the chopped tomatoes, along with the chilli flakes, cumin, paprika, sugar and lemon juice and simmer for a further 5–7 minutes until it starts to reduce. Now stir in the spinach and allow to wilt down for a couple of minutes.

Make 4 evenly spaced wells in the tomato mixture and crack one egg into each. Season well with salt and pepper and cover the frying pan with a lid. Cook for 10 minutes, or until the egg whites are firm but the yolks still runny, and serve straight away.

Tips & Tweaks

- You can prepare this in advance, or the night before. Just prepare the tomato mixture, but stop before adding the spinach. When you're ready to cook, reheat, then continue with the recipe, adding the spinach and eggs.
- If you are not dairy-free, serve with a tablespoon of Greek yogurt (1 tbsp = 15 cals).
- On a Regular Day, serve this with a wholemeal pitta bread (1 pitta = 145 cals) or a homemade flatbread (p. 156; 1 flatbread = 100 cals) to soak up the delicious sauce.

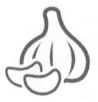

Power-through Porridges

I almost feel silly giving you a porridge recipe. I'm sure you already know how to make it, but this is all about the variations. If you are in need of something a bit decadent but still want to keep it healthy, then these little bowls of bliss are just what the doctor ordered. You can use non-dairy milk, if you prefer.

Quantity/serves: 1

Calories per serving (plain): 256

Prep time: **5 mins**

Cooking time: **6 mins**

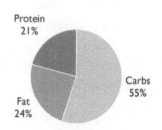

☒ Vegan   ☑ Lacto-Ovo Vegetarian

☒ Dairy-Free   ☑ Gluten-Free (use GF oats)

Ingredients

Plain
40g jumbo oats
200ml semi-skimmed milk
a pinch of salt

Variations

- **Banana, Coconut & Brown Sugar (321 cals):** Top with 50g thinly sliced banana, 1 tsp brown sugar and 1 tbsp light coconut milk.
- **Cinnamon, Walnuts & Honey (346 cals):** Top with ½ tsp ground cinnamon, 10g chopped walnuts (about 4 halves) and 1 tsp honey.
- **Peanut Choc Chip (347 cals):** Stir in 2 tsp (10g) dark chocolate chips and 1 tsp crunchy peanut butter.

- **Coconut Choc Chip (355 cals):** Stir in 2 tsp (10g) dark chocolate chips and 1 tbsp unsweetened desiccated coconut.
- **Malt Choc Chip (359 cals):** Stir in 2 tsp (10g) dark chocolate chips and 1 tbsp Horlicks or other malted drink powder.

Method

Place the oats, milk and salt in a saucepan and cook over a low heat, stirring frequently, for 6 minutes or until it reaches the desired consistency – you can add a little water if it gets too thick. Remove from the heat and add your chosen variation ingredients. Serve immediately.

Simple Smoothie Bowl

If you've never made a smoothie bowl before, you're in for a treat. This quick and healthy crowd-pleaser is simplicity itself: just put everything in a blender or NutriBullet and the work is done for you.

Quantity/serves: 1

Calories per serving: 284

Prep time: 10 mins

Cooking time: 0 mins

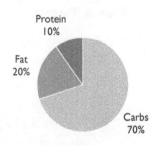

☒ Vegan   ☑ Lacto-Ovo Vegetarian

☒ Dairy-Free   ☑ Gluten-Free (assuming the granola is GF)

Ingredients

100g mixed frozen berries

1 small, ripe banana

2 tbsp Greek yogurt

2 tbsp semi-skimmed milk or light coconut milk

1 tbsp My Go-to Granola (p. 89) or shop-bought granola

1 tsp chia seeds

2 tsp unsweetened desiccated coconut

50g chopped fresh fruit (such as strawberries, blueberries, raspberries, mango, papaya or fresh figs)

Method

Put the frozen berries, banana, yogurt and milk in a blender and whizz together to produce a smoothie consistency. Pour into a bowl, leaving enough space for the toppings. Arrange the granola, chia seeds, coconut and chopped fruit in lines on the top, and enjoy.

Tips & Tweaks

- If you have ripe bananas, you can chop them up and freeze them: they'll be perfect to use in this recipe.
- You can use any combination of frozen fruit; mango and strawberry is also good.
- Adjust the toppings to suit family preferences. At the weekend, why not have a toppings 'buffet' so everyone can choose their own?

Mexican Breakfast Bowl

I have called this a Mexican Breakfast Bowl simply because it uses tomatoes, avocado, jalapeños and lime juice – some of my favourite ingredients – all in one bowl.

Quantity/serves: 2

Calories per serving: 312

Prep time: 10 mins

Cooking time: 5 mins

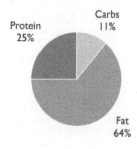

Protein 25%
Carbs 11%
Fat 64%

☒ Vegan   ☑ Lacto-Ovo Vegetarian

☒ Dairy-Free   ☑ Gluten-Free

Ingredients

    4 eggs, whisked
    a pinch of salt
    a pinch of freshly ground black pepper
    1 tomato, diced
    ½ avocado, peeled, stoned and sliced
    2 tbsp jalapeños, from a jar
    50g grated Cheddar
    juice of 1 lime

Method

Place a large, non-stick frying pan over a low heat. Pour the whisked eggs into the pan and season well with salt and pepper. Gently fold the eggs over a few times until scrambled.

Divide the eggs between two bowls and arrange the tomato, avocado and jalapeños on top. Scatter over the grated cheese, drizzle over a little lime juice and serve.

Tips & Tweaks

- Do the chopping and grating the night before (apart from the avocado, which will go brown) so you can just scramble the eggs and whack it all in a bowl in the morning.
- If you prefer to divide your 800 Light Day calories into two rather than three meals, this is a great choice for a balanced and filling brunch.
- On a Regular Day when you have more calories to play with, you can go off-piste – try different cheeses, other veggies, seeds, nuts or any leftovers you might have in the fridge.

Brekkie in a Hurry

Now I don't usually 'do' smoothies, as it's easier to just eat the fruit whole, but from time to time a quick blitz-up in the blender is a good way to get some nutrition in your belly – plus, kids love them. I've kept this flexible on the fruit front so you can chuck in whatever you have in the freezer.

Quantity/serves: 1

Calories per serving: 317

Prep time: 5 mins

Cooking time: 0 mins

☒ Vegan   ☑ Lacto-Ovo Vegetarian

☒ Dairy-Free   ☑ Gluten-Free (use GF oats)

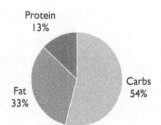

Protein 13%

Fat 33%

Carbs 54%

Ingredients

2 tbsp rolled oats

100g frozen fruit (blueberries, raspberries, cherries or mixed berries)

½ ripe banana, peeled

1 tbsp peanut or almond butter

100ml semi-skimmed milk

a few ice cubes

Method

Place the oats in the bottom of a blender and pulse a few times until finely ground. Add the frozen fruit, banana, nut butter, milk and ice cubes and blend on high until smooth and creamy, stopping to scrape down the blender as needed. If it's a bit too thick, add a small splash of water and blend again. Serve straight away.

Tips & Tweaks

- You can substitute nut milk or light coconut milk for the semi-skimmed milk to make a non-dairy version.
- You can freeze the other half of the banana to use another day.

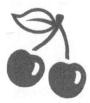

Quick Breakfast Assemblies

Often you simply don't have time to cook anything in the morning, but don't be tempted to just grab a bowl of cereal. I've come up with some really easy breakfast assemblies that are a much more nourishing way to start the day.

Crispbread Crackers with Smoked Salmon, Cream Cheese, Red Onion & Lemon Juice

Serves: 1

Calories per serving: 180

Fat: 32%   Protein: 30%   Carbs: 38%

Ingredients

> 2 crispbread crackers
> 1 tbsp light cream cheese
> 50g smoked salmon (2 slices)
> a few thin slices of red onion
> a squeeze of fresh lemon juice
> a pinch of freshly ground black pepper

Method

Spread the crackers with the cream cheese and place a slice of smoked salmon on top of each. Sprinkle over the thin red onion slices, and finish with a squeeze of lemon juice and a little black pepper.

Oatcakes with Tomato, Avocado & Feta

Serves: 1

Calories per serving: 268

Fat: 59%   Protein: 11%   Carbs: 30%

Ingredients

> 2 oatcakes
> 2 slices of tomato
> ¼ ripe avocado, peeled, stoned and sliced
> 25g feta cheese
> freshly chopped herbs or chives (optional)

Method

Top each oatcake with a slice of tomato, then cover with avocado slices and crumble over the feta cheese. If you have any fresh herbs or chives, these can be sprinkled over the top for added flavour.

Greek Yogurt, Blueberries, Lemon Curd and Chopped Walnuts

Serves: 1

Calories per serving: 210

Fat: 37%   Protein: 23%   Carbs: 40%

Ingredients

> 100g Greek yogurt
> 1 tbsp lemon curd
> 50g fresh blueberries (or other berries)
> 4 walnut halves, chopped

Method

Place the yogurt in a bowl and swirl in the lemon curd. Top with the berries and sprinkle over the chopped walnuts.

Some other Quick Breakfast Assemblies under 250 calories:

- 2 crispbread crackers, 100g cottage cheese and 1 sliced pear.

- 1 slice of wholegrain toast, topped with 1 scrambled egg and 1 slice of ham.

- 1 soft-boiled egg with 1 slice of seedy toast for dipping, and 1 tangerine.

- ½ toasted cinnamon bagel, topped with 1 tsp peanut butter and some slices of banana.

- 1 slice of toasted sourdough bread, topped with ½ medium-sized avocado and some chopped tomatoes.

- 3 tbsp Greek yogurt, topped with 2 tbsp granola and a handful of berries.

- A simple smoothie made with 120ml semi-skimmed milk, 50g Greek yogurt, 100g frozen berries and 1 tsp maple syrup.

- 2 eggs whisked together and fried in a pan with a handful of spinach leaves, topped with 20g grated Cheddar cheese.

- A few sliced mushrooms and 1 sliced tomato, fried in a pan with 1 tsp olive oil, a pinch of dried chilli flakes (optional), salt and pepper. Serve in a wholegrain pitta bread with 1 tbsp Greek yogurt.

Stuff on Toast

If you've ever been on a low-carb diet, the thought of 'stuff on toast' might be a bit scary, but good-quality wholegrain bread is good for you. In fact, a supply of complex carbs is important for all kinds of reasons in midlife, one of which is hormone balance. Plus, toast is totally delicious. You will notice I don't butter the toast: 1 teaspoon of butter adds 35 calories, so it's best to leave it out on a Light Day, but if it's a Regular Day, go ahead if you like. Also, I have given these as one-slice options; on a Regular Day, you could go for two slices, but I usually find that one is enough, especially if I have some fresh fruit with it as well.

QUICK STUFF ON TOAST

Nut Butter, Banana & Cinnamon

Calories: 257 Fat: 32% Protein: 15% Carbs: 53%

Toast 1 slice of good-quality, wholegrain bread. Spread with 1 tbsp nut butter, cover with slices of banana and dust over a little cinnamon to taste.

Avocado, Parmesan & Lemon Juice

Calories: 229 Fat: 44% Protein: 17% Carbs: 39%

Toast 1 slice of good-quality, wholegrain bread. Mash on ¼ avocado, grate over 10g Parmesan cheese and finish with a squeeze of lemon juice.

Coronation Hummus, Feta & Spring Onions

Calories: 166   Fat: 27%   Protein: 19%   Carbs: 54%

Toast 1 slice of good-quality, wholegrain bread. Spread with 1 tbsp Coronation Hummus (p. 126) or shop-bought hummus, crumble over 10g feta cheese and scatter over 1 chopped spring onion.

Cream Cheese, Smoked Salmon, Lemon & Red Onion

Calories: 184   Fat: 27%   Protein: 30%   Carbs: 43%

Toast 1 slice of good-quality, wholegrain bread. Spread with 1 tbsp light cream cheese, cover with a palm-sized piece of smoked salmon, squeeze over a little lemon juice and top with a few thin slices of red onion. Finish with a grind of black pepper.

Yeast Extract, Cucumber & Cheddar

Calories: 165   Fat: 27%   Protein: 24%   Carbs: 49%

Toast 1 slice of good-quality, wholegrain bread. Spread with 1 tsp yeast extract (or to taste), cover with slices of cucumber and grate over 10g Cheddar.

SLOWER STUFF ON TOAST

Sautéed Leeks, Dijon Mustard & Mature Cheddar

Calories: 183   Fat: 26%   Protein: 19%   Carbs: 55%

Heat 1 tsp oil in a frying pan. Add about 50g thinly sliced leek, season and sauté gently for around 5 minutes, until soft. Toast 1 slice of good-quality, wholegrain bread. Spread thinly with Dijon mustard and place the leeks on top. Cover with 10g of grated mature Cheddar.

Sautéed Paprika Peppers, Goat's Cheese & Egg

Calories: 286   Fat: 47%   Protein: 22%   Carbs: 31%

Thinly slice ½ red pepper and place in a hot frying pan with 1 tsp oil and ½ tsp paprika. Sauté for 5 minutes until soft and starting to brown. Remove from the pan, then fry the egg in the same pan. Meanwhile, toast 1 slice of good-quality, wholegrain bread. Top the toast with the peppers and egg, then finish with 20g soft goat's cheese.

Boiled Egg, Avocado & Watercress

Calories: 254   Fat: 46%   Protein: 19%   Carbs: 35%

Place an egg in a pan of boiling water and cook (5 minutes for soft-boiled; 7 minutes for medium-boiled; 10 minutes for hard-boiled). Run under cold water and peel. Toast 1 slice of good-quality, wholegrain bread and mash on ¼ avocado. Place the egg on top. If soft- or medium-boiled, gently open up; if hard-boiled, slice. Season well, then snip over some watercress with a pair of scissors.

Roast Tomatoes & Spicy Seeds

Calories: 196   Fat: 36%   Protein: 15%   Carbs: 49%

Preheat the oven to 170°C/gas mark 3½. Place 10 cherry tomatoes in a small baking tray, drizzle with 1 tsp olive oil, season and bake for 10 minutes until blistered and soft. Toast 1 slice of good-quality, wholegrain bread. Mash the cooked tomatoes on top, then sprinkle over 1 tsp Spicy Seeds Topper (p. 122).

Mushrooms, Wilted Spinach & Chilli Flakes

Calories: 167   Fat: 31%   Protein: 19%   Carbs: 50%

Heat 1 tsp butter in a frying pan. Add a handful of spinach leaves and a handful of sliced mushrooms, season well and sauté gently for a few minutes until softened. Meanwhile, toast 1 slice of good-quality, wholegrain bread. Place the mushrooms and spinach on top and sprinkle over a few dried chilli flakes.

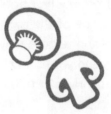

MEALS BY CALORIE COUNT

Spicy Seeds Topper

This recipe is adapted from my first book, *The Midlife Kitchen*, because it proved to be one of the most popular! It's a big pop of health-boosting taste and texture that you can use to jump-start eggs, salads, soups and wraps. I call it my flavour saviour. 1 teaspoon of this mix contains just 20 calories, so it's brilliant for jazzing up Light Day meals.

Quantity/serves: n/a

Calories per tsp: 20

Prep time: 5 mins

Cooking time: 5 mins

☑ Vegan   ☑ Lacto-Ovo Vegetarian

☑ Dairy-Free   ☑ Gluten-Free

Protein 14%   Carbs 11%   Fat 75%

Ingredients

100g mixed seeds (such as pumpkin, sunflower, flax or sesame)
2 tsp extra-virgin olive oil
1 tsp ground turmeric
1 tsp ground cumin
1 tsp ground coriander
½ tsp dried chilli flakes
a good pinch of salt
a good pinch of freshly ground black pepper

Method

Place a large frying pan over a medium heat. Add the mixed seeds and dry-fry for several minutes until they start to colour and pop. In a bowl, mix together the oil and spices. Add the seeds and mix well to combine. Finally, season to taste. This will keep for up to 2 weeks in an airtight container.

Tips & Tweaks

- I often make double quantities of this because I use it up so quickly.
- You'll be amazed how often you can use this mix to add pep to a dish, so keep it to hand on the countertop and sprinkle away.

Pintopeño Dip

I'm a big fan of a portmanteau, particularly when the two things involved also go so well together flavour-wise: in this case, pinto beans and jalapeños. It's always a good idea to have some kind of homemade dip in the fridge for healthy snacking, or as a filler for a lunchtime wrap.

Quantity/serves: 750g (15 × 50g servings)

Calories per servings: 44

Prep time: 10 mins

Cooking time: 0 mins

☑ Vegan   ☑ Lacto-Ovo Vegetarian

☑ Dairy-Free   ☑ Gluten-Free

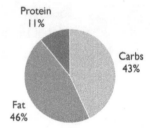

Protein 11%
Carbs 43%
Fat 46%

Ingredients

400g can pinto beans, drained and rinsed
1 garlic clove, finely grated
1 tbsp extra-virgin olive oil
1–2 tbsp jalapeños, from a jar (add more
   if you like it hotter)
1 ripe avocado, peeled, stoned and chopped
3 ripe tomatoes, chopped
juice of ½ lemon (or add more to taste)
a handful of coriander leaves, freshly chopped
a pinch of salt
a pinch of freshly ground black pepper

Method

Place all the ingredients in a food processor or blender. Blend on a medium speed for about 20 seconds, then use a spatula to scrape down the sides of the bowl. You can blend it a little more for a smoother dip, or leave it a bit chunkier if you prefer. Transfer to an airtight container to chill in the fridge.

Tips & Tweaks

- This can be made in advance and kept in the fridge for a few days.
- For a Light Day lunch, spread this in a wholemeal pitta with veggies (1 wholemeal pitta, 1 serving of dip and a handful of salad veg = 200 cals) or dollop some over mixed leaves with some canned sweetcorn for a lovely Mexican-inspired salad (100g salad leaves, 1 serving of dip and 200g canned sweetcorn = 200 cals).
- This goes well with veggie sticks or toasted pitta triangles as a snack on a Regular Day.

Coronation Hummus

This is my absolute favourite hummus variation – and that's saying something, because I have tried many, many riffs on this healthy classic. The trick is to keep the spicing subtle but discernible: a hit of background heat that isn't too overpowering.

Quantity/serves: 350g (7 × 50g servings)

Calories per servings: 67

Prep time: 10 mins

Cooking time: 0 mins

☒ Vegan   ☑ Lacto-Ovo Vegetarian

☒ Dairy-Free   ☑ Gluten-Free

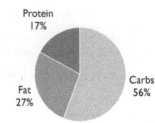

Protein 17%
Fat 27%
Carbs 56%

Ingredients

400g can chickpeas, drained and rinsed
1 tbsp Greek yogurt
1 tbsp tahini
1 garlic clove, peeled and crushed
1 large green chilli, deseeded and chopped
2 tbsp lemon juice
1 tsp ground cumin
1 tsp ground turmeric
1 tsp mild curry powder
a pinch of salt
a pinch of freshly ground black pepper

Method

Place all the ingredients in a food processor or blender. Blend on a low speed for about 30 seconds, then scrape down the sides of the blender with a spatula. Continue to blend on high for a couple of minutes. If the mixture seems too stiff, you can slowly add a little water (1 teaspoon at a time). You might have to stop and scrape down the sides again midway through. Transfer to an airtight container to chill in the fridge before serving. It will keep in the fridge for up to 3 days.

Tips & Tweaks

- You can make this in advance and keep it in the fridge until you're ready to eat: the flavour gets even better.
- Excellent used in a wrap (see Chicken & Hummus Romaine Wraps on p. 196).
- Serve with some veggie sticks for a healthy snack on a Regular Day.
- I serve this as a dinner party 'nibble' with toasted wholemeal pittas cut into triangles.

Rich Tomato Sauce

We all need a good basic tomato sauce in our repertoire, and this is mine. The secret to the flavour is in the slow cooking of the onions first. This sauce is used in my recipes for Italian Aubergines (p. 176) and Easy Spinach & Ricotta Wholewheat Cannelloni (p. 220). You can also use it to make a Bolognese, or freestyle with veggies, prawns, herbs and spices.

Quantity/serves: 10 × 100g servings

Calories per serving: 79

Prep time: **10 mins**

Cooking time: **60 mins**

☑ Vegan   ☑ Lacto-Ovo Vegetarian

☑ Dairy-Free   ☑ Gluten-Free

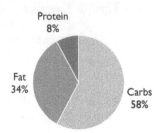

Protein 8%

Fat 34%

Carbs 58%

Ingredients

    2 tbsp olive oil
    1 onion, finely diced
    2 garlic cloves, crushed
    2 tsp dried oregano
    3 × 400g cans good-quality chopped tomatoes
    1 tsp brown sugar
    2 tsp red wine vinegar
    a pinch of salt
    a pinch of freshly ground black pepper
    a handful of fresh basil, chopped (optional)

Method

Heat the oil in a large saucepan over a low heat and add the onion. Cook gently for about 10 minutes, until softened and translucent but not browned – you may need to add a little water if it gets too dry. Stir in the garlic and cook for another 2 minutes. Add the oregano, tomatoes, sugar and vinegar and bring to the boil. Check the seasoning, add salt and pepper to taste, then simmer gently for 45 minutes, adding the chopped basil 5 minutes before the end (if using). Leave the sauce chunky or blitz in the food processor if you prefer it smooth.

Tips & Tweaks

- This is best made in advance as the flavour improves with time, so make a big batch on a rainy day and keep it in meal-sized portions in the freezer.
- You could also use this sauce as a base for a veggie or meat lasagne. Use wholewheat lasagne sheets for more fibre.

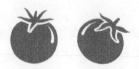

Quick Smoked Mackerel & Butter Bean Fishcakes

Fishcakes are the ultimate in 'chuck together' dinners and everyone loves them. Here, because I've used packs of smoked mackerel and a tin of butter beans, they're even quicker to prepare – no potato boiling required. Don't worry that these might be too fishy if you have younger kids: they really aren't, and in any case, the kids will probably cover them in ketchup anyway!

Quantity/serves: makes 10 fishcakes

Calories per fishcake: 99

Prep time: **15 mins**

Cooking time: **8 mins**

☒ Vegan   ☒ Lacto-Ovo Vegetarian

☑ Dairy-Free   ☑ Gluten-Free (use GF flour)

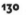

Protein 36%

Carbs 26%

Fat 38%

Ingredients

 1 small handful of fresh flat-leaf parsley
 3 spring onions, roughly chopped
 400g can butter beans, drained and rinsed
 2 smoked mackerel fillets, skin removed, roughly flaked
 juice of ½ lemon
 1 egg
 a good pinch of salt
 a good pinch of freshly ground black pepper
 wholemeal flour (or gluten-free flour), to coat
 2 tsp neutral oil (or spray oil), for frying

Method

Place the parsley and spring onions in a food processor and pulse a couple of times. Add the beans and process on a low speed until the beans and greens are well combined. Add the flaked mackerel, lemon juice, egg, salt and pepper and pulse to form a soft mixture. If the mixture is too wet to handle, add a tablespoon of the flour. Taking a small handful of the mixture (around 45g), roll it into a ball and then flatten slightly. Put a few tablespoons of the flour on to a large plate, then place the fishcake in the flour, turning so that both sides are well coated. Repeat this process until you have 10 coated fishcakes.

Place a large frying pan over a medium heat and add the oil. Swirl the oil around to coat the base, then place the fishcakes in the pan. Depending on the size of the pan, you may have to work in batches. Reduce the heat if they are browning too quickly. Cook for around 5 minutes (or until golden), then flip over and cook for another 5 minutes on the other side. Serve immediately.

Tips & Tweaks

- These can be prepared in advance up to the point of frying, then frozen until needed. Be sure to defrost thoroughly prior to cooking.
- Mix together equal quantities of Dijon mustard and Greek yogurt for a lovely dipping sauce (1 tbsp = 15 cals). Alternatively, serve with a little horseradish sauce (1 tsp = 20 cals).
- Serve with blanched green beans on a Light Day.
- I've supplied the calories per fishcake, so you can decide how many to have depending on whether it's a Light Day or a Regular Day.

'They'll Never Know' Veggie Ragu

This is my version of a veggie Bolognese sauce: it's perfect with spaghetti, obviously, but also a good alternative to meat sauce in a lasagne. The secret meat stand-in here is chestnut mushrooms, blitzed in the food processor to resemble minced beef – but don't worry, it doesn't taste overwhelmingly of mushrooms. It's just rich and tomatoey, like a proper ragu should be.

Quantity/serves: 6

Calories per serving (sauce only): 99

Prep time: 10 mins

Cooking time: 60 mins

☑ Vegan   ☑ Lacto-Ovo Vegetarian

☑ Dairy-Free   ☑ Gluten-Free

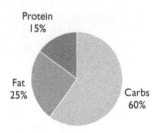

Protein 15%
Fat 25%
Carbs 60%

Ingredients

1 red onion, chopped
2 garlic cloves, roughly chopped
1 tbsp extra-virgin olive oil
250g chestnut mushrooms
700ml passata
50g dried red lentils
1 tsp dried oregano (or mixed dried herbs)
1 tsp brown sugar
a pinch of salt
a pinch of freshly ground black pepper

Method

Place the onion and garlic in a food processor and blitz to a fine pulp. Heat the oil in a large saucepan over a low heat and add the onion and garlic mixture. Fry gently for a couple of minutes to soften. In the meantime, put the mushrooms in the food processor and blitz into small pieces. Now add the mushrooms to the pan and continue to fry for another 2–3 minutes. Pour in the passata, then rinse out the bottle with water (fill it about three-quarters full) and add the tomatoey water to the pan, too. Add the lentils, oregano and sugar, and season well with salt and pepper. Now reduce the heat right down, place a lid loosely on the pan and simmer for 1 hour, stirring occasionally. Add more water during the cooking process if the sauce is getting too thick.

Tips & Tweaks

- This recipe really does require a food processor – you can dice the onions and mushrooms by hand, but you won't be able to get them as fine.
- Serve with wholewheat spaghetti (100g cooked weight = 124 cals) and a leafy salad.

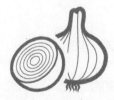

Beetroot, Carrot & Apple Slaw

This is such a simple salad, and it has the advantage of actually tasting a bit better when it's made in advance, so it can sit happily in the fridge for a day or so. Beetroot, carrot and apple are natural bedfellows, while the onion adds tang and the mint brings the whole thing alive. This is sure to become a favourite.

Quantity/serves: 4

Calories per serving: 122

Prep time: 10 mins

Cooking time: 0 mins

☒ Vegan   ☑ Lacto-Ovo Vegetarian

☑ Dairy-Free   ☑ Gluten-Free

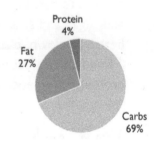

Protein 4%
Fat 27%
Carbs 69%

Ingredients

200g carrots, peeled
1 apple, cored, skin on
200g raw beetroot, peeled
100g red onions, finely sliced
a small handful of mint leaves, chopped

For the dressing
1 tbsp extra-virgin olive oil
juice of 1 lemon
1 tbsp runny honey
a pinch of salt
a pinch of freshly ground black pepper

Method

Using the medium-sized grater attachment in your food processor, grate the carrot, apple and beetroot. Transfer to a large bowl and toss together with the sliced red onions and mint leaves.

In a small bowl, mix together the dressing ingredients, then pour over the salad. Toss well to combine.

Tips & Tweaks

- This is best done using the grater attachment in your food processor – if you're grating by hand instead, add 10 minutes to the prep time.
- This tastes even better if you leave it to sit in the fridge for an hour or two, or even overnight – give it another good mix before serving.
- Have this on its own as a Light Day meal with some cooked chicken breast for protein (100g = 165 cals) or as a side dish on a Regular Day.

Broccoli, Bacon & Cheddar Burgers

Well, OK, these aren't really burgers, but I despise the word 'patty', so burgers it is. These have had very positive feedback, so I'm excited to share them with you. Make a double batch – they work for brekkie, too.

Quantity/serves: makes 10 burgers

Calories per serving (3 burgers): 160

Prep time: 15 mins

Cooking time: 15 mins

☒ Vegan   ☒ Lacto-Ovo Vegetarian

☒ Dairy-Free ☒ Gluten-Free

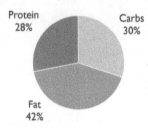

Protein 28%
Carbs 30%
Fat 42%

Ingredients

1 head (approx. 250g) broccoli
35g fresh brown breadcrumbs
50g back bacon, any excess fat trimmed, chopped
½ large onion, finely diced
50g mature Cheddar cheese, grated
a small handful of fresh flat-leaf parsley, chopped
1 egg, whisked
a pinch of salt
a pinch of freshly ground black pepper

Method

Preheat the oven to 200°C/gas mark 6 and line a baking tray with baking parchment.

Fill a large saucepan with water and bring to the boil. Place the broccoli head in (whole) and cook for 3 minutes. Take off the heat and immediately immerse the broccoli head in cold water, then pat dry with a tea towel and chop the broccoli up into small pieces, or pulse in a food processor. Place the chopped broccoli in a large bowl, and add the breadcrumbs.

Place a frying pan over a medium heat and add the bacon and onion. Fry for 2–3 minutes, until the bacon and onion are cooked but not browned. Add the bacon and onion to the bowl with the broccoli and breadcrumbs, then add the cheese, parsley, whisked egg, and salt and pepper. Use your hands to combine all the ingredients, kneading everything together to make a burger-like mixture. Take handfuls of the mixture, form them into burger shapes and place on the lined baking tray. This recipe will make 10 burgers. Bake for 15 minutes and serve.

Tips & Tweaks

- Whizz up a thick slice of brown bread in a food processor to make the breadcrumbs.
- The mixture seems like it will fall apart, but don't worry – as it cooks, the egg and cheese bind everything together.
- If you like heat, a little sriracha sauce works a treat with these, or you can sprinkle over some dried chilli flakes.
- A portion is only 160 calories, so you can afford to add a few extras, even on a Light Day. I love these with a poached egg on top (1 egg = 75 cals).

Green Lentil, Tomato & Watercress Soup

ANDI stands for Aggregate Nutrient Density Index, a scoring system that rates foods on a scale from 1 to 1,000, based on their nutrient content. And guess what's right at the top? Watercress. No further reasons needed, then, to include it in this nourishing and delicious soup.

Quantity/serves: 3

Calories per serving: 164

Prep time: 15 mins

Cooking time: 20 mins

☑ Vegan   ☑ Lacto-Ovo Vegetarian

☑ Dairy-Free   ☑ Gluten-Free

Protein 16%

Fat 29%

Carbs 55%

Ingredients

1 tbsp extra-virgin olive oil
1 small red onion, finely diced
2 garlic cloves, crushed
1 tsp ground cumin
1 tsp ground coriander
1 tsp ground turmeric
200g (½ can) chopped tomatoes
500ml vegetable stock, made from a cube
400g can green lentils in water, drained
1 carrot, peeled and grated
a pinch of sea salt
a pinch of freshly ground black pepper
a handful of watercress leaves, picked and chopped
a squeeze of fresh lemon juice

Method

Heat the oil in a large saucepan over a medium heat. Add the onion, garlic, cumin, coriander and turmeric, and gently fry for around 5 minutes, adding a drop of water if they start to stick. Add the tomatoes, stock, lentils and carrot. Bring to the boil, then simmer for 10 minutes until everything has softened. Season with salt and pepper. Transfer the soup to a blender and pulse a few times, or use a stick blender. Aim for a fairly thick, coarsely textured soup. Stir in the chopped watercress leaves and a squeeze of fresh lemon juice. Heat through for 5 minutes before serving.

Tips & Tweaks

- If using dried lentils, increase the simmering time to 30 minutes and add some extra water, as the lentils will keep absorbing it.
- Swirl in some Greek yogurt just before serving (1 tbsp = 15 cals).
- Serve with a slice of wholegrain bread (1 slice = 100 cals).

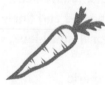

Seafood Stew with Fennel & Turmeric

The simplicity of this stew belies the complex flavours that develop when it is left to, well, stew. There's a lazy magic about ingredients left bubbling over a low flame, slowly transforming themselves into a pan of rich deliciousness.

Quantity/serves: 4

Calories per portion: 166

Prep time: **15 mins**

Cooking time: **45 mins**

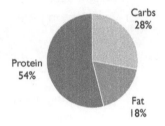

Carbs 28%

Protein 54%

Fat 18%

☒ Vegan   ☒ Lacto-Ovo Vegetarian

☑ Dairy-Free   ☑ Gluten-Free

Ingredients

1 tsp olive oil
2 garlic cloves, finely grated
1 tsp fennel seeds
1 small fennel bulb, finely sliced
2 small carrots, peeled and finely sliced
2 spring onions or 1 small leek,
    finely sliced
1 tsp ground turmeric
400g can chopped tomatoes
500ml vegetable stock, made from
    a cube
a pinch of salt
a pinch of freshly ground black pepper
250g firm white fish fillet (such as cod), cut into
    large cubes
150g raw prawns, shelled

a handful of fresh flat-leaf parsley, chopped
juice of ½ lemon
a few drops of hot sauce (optional) to taste

Method

Heat the oil in a large saucepan over a low heat and add the garlic and fennel seeds. Fry for a minute or so, then add the fennel, carrots and spring onions/leek. Cook for around 5 minutes until the vegetables begin to soften, adding in a little water if it gets too dry, then add the turmeric, tomatoes and 400ml of the stock. Season well. Simmer, very gently, for 30 minutes until the contents of the pan have reduced right down.

Add the fish and prawns and top up with the rest of the stock. Stir well and simmer for a further 15 minutes. Stir in the parsley, squeeze over the lemon, add the hot sauce (if you like a bit of a kick) and serve.

Tips & Tweaks

- This is a good one to make in advance, as it tastes even better the next day.
- This stew is crying out for something to soak up the juices – some nutty brown rice is just the job (100g cooked weight = 110 cals), with some green beans on the side (100g = 31 cals).

Roast Romaine with Feta Drizzle

I'm a big fan of roasting vegetables: it improves their flavour no end and requires very little effort. I also love feta, which has bags of taste but is lower in fat than many other cheeses. I recommend using the Spicy Seeds Topper (p. 122) to give this more crunch and a hit of heat.

Quantity/serves: 2

Calories per portion: 172

Prep time: 15 mins

Cooking time: 15 mins

☒ Vegan   ☑ Lacto-Ovo Vegetarian

☒ Dairy-Free   ☑ Gluten-Free

Protein 20%
Carbs 26%
Fat 54%

Ingredients

1 large romaine lettuce (or you can use 2 baby gems)
1 tsp extra-virgin olive oil
70g feta cheese
1 tbsp Greek yogurt
a small handful of mint leaves, chopped
1 tbsp lemon juice
a good pinch of freshly ground black pepper

Method

Preheat the oven to 200°C/gas mark 6.

Split the lettuce lengthways from tip to root. Rub the olive oil all over the lettuce halves and place them on a baking tray, cut-side up. Roast for 10 minutes, until softened and just starting to brown at the edges.

Meanwhile, place all the other ingredients in a blender and pulse until fully combined. The mixture should be fairly runny, so it can be 'drizzled' – add a drop of water or a little more yogurt if needed.

Remove the lettuce from the oven, arrange on a plate and drizzle over the feta mixture to serve.

Tips & Tweaks

- This is a super Light Day lunch or an excellent side dish to some grilled lamb cutlets on a Regular Day.
- Sprinkle over some Spicy Seeds Topper (p. 122; 1 tsp = 20 cals).

Broccerino Soup

When we are focused on eating with awareness, it's helpful to have something really healthy and tasty ready to eat at a moment's notice. So, make a load of this soup, stick it in the fridge and you're good to go!

Quantity/serves: 4

Calories per portion: 173

Prep time: **5 mins**

Cooking time: **15 mins**

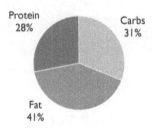

☒ Vegan   ☒ Lacto-Ovo Vegetarian

☒ Dairy-Free   ☑ Gluten-Free

Ingredients

> 1 tsp olive oil
> 1 red onion, diced
> 2 garlic cloves, finely grated
> 500ml vegetable stock, made from a cube
> 2 heads (approx. 500g) of broccoli, chopped
> 500ml semi-skimmed milk
> 1 heaped tsp smooth Dijon mustard
> 50g Pecorino (or Parmesan) cheese, finely grated
> a pinch of salt
> a pinch of freshly ground black pepper

Method

Place the oil in a large saucepan over a low heat. Add the onion and garlic and fry gently for 2–3 minutes. Add the stock and then the broccoli. Add the milk, making sure the broccoli is well covered. Stir in the mustard and cheese, then bring to the boil and simmer gently for 15–20 minutes until the broccoli is tender. Allow to cool a little before blending to a smooth consistency in a blender or food processor, or with a stick blender. Season with salt and pepper to taste. Add a little water to loosen if it's too thick, then reheat and serve.

Tips & Tweaks

- I love to swirl yogurt into most things and this is no exception (1 tbsp = 15 cals).
- This is a pretty filling soup, so just having it on its own is fine on a Light Day. Add a slice of crusty bread on a Regular Day (1 slice = 100 cals).
- This soup will keep for 3–4 days in the fridge.

Carrot, Lemon & Ginger Soup

Carrot and coriander soup is a classic combination, but the real genius here is the base of red lentils and lemon, which give it a brilliant texture and taste lift. Another great addition is the fresh ginger, which complements the sweet carrot so well.

Quantity/serves: 2

Calories per portion: 186

Prep time: **10 mins**

Cooking time: **20 mins**

☑ Vegan   ☑ Lacto-Ovo Vegetarian

☑ Dairy-Free   ☑ Gluten-Free

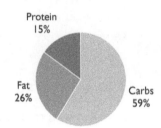

Protein 15%

Fat 26%

Carbs 59%

Ingredients

30g dried red lentils

zest of ½ lemon

2cm piece of fresh root ginger, peeled and finely sliced

300g carrots, peeled and chopped

½ onion, roughly chopped

500ml vegetable stock, made from a cube

leaves from 2 fresh coriander sprigs, plus extra to serve

100ml light coconut milk

a pinch of salt

a pinch of freshly ground black pepper

Method

Put the lentils, lemon zest and ginger into a food processor and pulse to combine. You will need to pulse and then scrape down the sides a few times. Add the carrots and onion and pulse again until everything is coarsely chopped.

Transfer the mixture to a large saucepan. Use a splash of the stock to rinse out the food processor bowl and pour that into the saucepan, followed by the rest of the stock. Place the pan over a medium heat and bring to the boil, then reduce the heat to low and simmer for 15 minutes. Add the coriander leaves and coconut milk and stir well. Return the soup to the food processor and blend on high until smooth. Taste and season with salt and pepper accordingly. Add a little water to loosen if required. Return to the saucepan to warm through, then serve, topped with a few more coriander leaves.

Tips & Tweaks

- Blitzing the ingredients in the food processor first reduces the overall cooking time and maximises the flavour released from the lemon and ginger.
- Top with a pinch of dried chilli flakes if you like a bit of a kick.
- Serve with some wholegrain bread (1 slice = 100 cals) or a couple of oatcakes (1 oatcake = 45 cals).

Roast Cod with Basil Sauce & Cherry Tomatoes

I prefer to cook fish in the oven, because if you pan-fry it, you end up with a fishy aroma lingering long after you've finished your meal. Cod roasts really well and basil and tomatoes are a classic and delicious combination.

Quantity/serves: 4

Calories per portion: 186

Prep time: 10 mins

Cooking time: 15–20 mins

☒ Vegan   ☒ Lacto-Ovo Vegetarian

☑ Dairy-Free   ☑ Gluten-Free

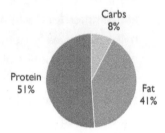

Carbs 8%

Protein 51%

Fat 41%

Ingredients

20 cherry tomatoes
1 tsp extra-virgin olive oil
4 cod fillets (approx. 140g each)
a good pinch of salt
a good pinch of freshly ground black pepper

For the basil sauce
50g basil leaves
2 tbsp extra-virgin olive oil
1 tbsp lemon juice
1 garlic clove, peeled and chopped

Method

Preheat the oven to 200°C/gas mark 6.

Place the cherry tomatoes in a baking dish. Drizzle over the 1 teaspoon extra-virgin olive oil and toss well. Place the cod fillets in the dish among the tomatoes.

To make the basil sauce, put the basil, oil, lemon juice and garlic in a blender or food processor and pulse repeatedly to blend to a pesto-like paste. You may have to use a spatula to scrape down the sides a few times. Spoon the basil mixture evenly over the cod, then sprinkle a good amount of salt and pepper all over the fish and tomatoes.

Place the dish in the hot oven and bake until the fish is opaque and flakes easily with a fork: this will take 15–20 minutes, depending on the thickness of the fillets. Serve straight from the dish.

Tips & Tweaks

- You can prep this in advance and keep in the fridge until it's time to roast.
- My favourite veg to go with this is lightly blanched asparagus (100g = 20 cals).
- On a Light Day, stick to fish and plenty of veg, but on a Regular Day, some boiled baby new potatoes tossed in a little butter and some chopped fresh herbs are a nice addition (100g = approx. 100 cals).

Potato, Leek & Fennel Soup with Stilton

This is comfort food of the highest order: filling, tasty and somewhat retro, it's everything you need to make Light Days a breeze. It's so low in calories that you can have it with a lovely slice of grainy bread and still come in under 300.

Quantity/serves: 4

Calories per serving: 191

Prep time: **15 mins**

Cooking time: **35 mins**

☑ Vegan (omit Stilton)

☑ Lacto-Ovo Vegetarian

☑ Dairy-Free (omit Stilton)   ☑ Gluten-Free

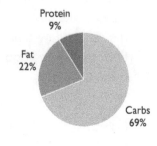

Protein 9%

Fat 22%

Carbs 69%

Ingredients

    2 tsp olive oil
    2 leeks, finely chopped
    1 small red onion, finely diced
    1 large potato, peeled and diced
    1 large fennel bulb, finely chopped
    1 litre vegetable stock, made from cubes
    a pinch of salt
    a pinch of freshly ground black pepper
    25g crumbled Stilton, to garnish (optional
       – omit for vegan/dairy-free option)

Method

Heat the oil in a large saucepan over a low heat. Add all the chopped vegetables and sweat for 5 minutes, then pour over enough stock to cover the vegetables and simmer gently for 30 minutes. Take off the heat and blend in a food processor or with a stick blender until smooth. If it's too thick, add any leftover stock or a little water and stir well. Season with salt and pepper to taste, and warm through before serving. Crumble over a little Stilton to garnish, if using.

Tips & Tweaks

- Reduce the prep time by using a food processor to chop up all the vegetables.
- If you're not making a vegan/dairy-free version, swirl in some Greek yogurt just before serving to give a nice, creamy tang (1 tbsp = 15 cals).

Spicy Roast Veg & Chickpeas with Mint & Yogurt

In the era BO (Before Ottolenghi) most of us probably would not have thought of pairing veggies, mint and yogurt, but now it seems as natural as, well, yogurt. If I'm really struggling for inspiration but I know I want to eat something healthy and filling, then roasting some vegetables is a good place to start. This particular combination is a favourite.

Quantity/serves: 4

Calories per portion: 191

Prep time: 10 mins

Cooking time: 35 mins

☒ Vegan   ☑ Lacto-Ovo Vegetarian

☒ Dairy-Free   ☑ Gluten-Free

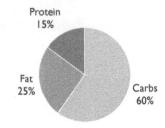

Protein 15%

Fat 25%

Carbs 60%

Ingredients

1 tbsp olive oil
½ tsp ground cumin
½ tsp ground coriander
½ tsp mixed spice (or cinnamon)
¼ tsp dried chilli flakes (optional)
a good pinch of salt
a good pinch of freshly ground black pepper
1 small butternut squash (approx. 500g), deseeded and cut into chunks (see Tips & Tweaks)
1 large red onion, cut into large chunks
1 lemon, quartered
100g cherry tomatoes

400g can chickpeas, drained and rinsed
a handful of mint leaves, picked and chopped if large
2 tbsp Greek yogurt

Method

Preheat the oven to 190°C/gas mark 5.

In a small bowl, mix together the oil, cumin, coriander, mixed spice or cinnamon and chilli flakes, if using, along with the salt and pepper. Place the squash and onion in a large roasting tin. Pour over the oil-and-spice mixture and stir to coat the vegetables well, then tuck the lemon wedges in among them. Roast in the oven for 20 minutes.

After 20 minutes, remove from the oven and add the tomatoes and chickpeas. Give everything a good stir, then roast for another 15 minutes. Remove from the oven and, when cool enough to handle, squeeze the roasted lemon wedges over the vegetables and chickpeas. Sprinkle over the mint leaves and serve with the Greek yogurt on the side, ready to spoon over.

Tips & Tweaks

- There's no need to peel the butternut squash: the skin goes lovely and soft when roasted.
- Add a sprinkle of pomegranate seeds for a final Ottolenghi-style flourish (100g = 83 cals).
- This is perfect as a Light Day lunch or as a side on a Regular Day.

Spinach & Parmesan Crustless Quiche

When you are watching the calories but really want some comfort food, this is just the ticket! All the goodness of eggs and spinach, but with no pastry to up the sat fat and calorie count. The perfect Light Day breakfast or brunch.

Quantity/serves: 4

Calories per serving: 196

Prep time: **10 mins**

Cooking time: **25 mins**

☒ Vegan   ☒ Lacto-Ovo Vegetarian

☒ Dairy-Free   ☑ Gluten-Free (use ground almonds)

Protein 28%
Carbs 24%
Fat 48%

Ingredients

4 eggs
300ml semi-skimmed milk
200g spinach leaves, washed
100g red onion, finely chopped
1 tsp olive oil
2 tbsp wholemeal flour (for GF, use ground almonds)
½ tsp dried chilli flakes (optional)
a pinch of salt
a pinch of freshly ground black pepper
50g Parmesan, grated

Method

Preheat the oven to 200°C/gas mark 6 and line a baking tin with baking parchment (see Tips & Tweaks).

Whisk together the eggs and milk in a jug. Place the spinach in a large frying pan over a low heat for a few minutes to wilt, then transfer to a bowl. Remove any excess water by squeezing the spinach with some kitchen roll – it needs to be as dry as possible. In the same pan, gently heat the olive oil and add the red onion. Fry for 2 minutes, then sprinkle the flour or ground almonds over the onions to coat. Add the onions to the bowl with the spinach.

Now pour the egg mixture into the bowl and add the chilli flakes, if using. Season well with salt and pepper and stir everything together. Pour the mixture into the prepared tin and top with the grated Parmesan. Bake for 25 minutes.

Leave to cool slightly, then lift out of the tin. Cut into 6 squares, then cut each square into 2 triangles. A serving is 3 triangles.

Tips & Tweaks

- To cook this, I use a deep, rectangular tin (approx. 20 × 15cm) and cover the entire interior with one piece of baking parchment. If you make sure the parchment comes up a little higher than the sides of the tin, then when the quiche is cooked and slightly cooled, you can just lift the whole thing out.
- This is lovely eaten warm, but it can also be kept in the fridge for up to 2 days, making it ideal for packed lunches and picnics. Some moisture can escape after a while, so store in an airtight container with a layer of kitchen roll underneath.
- Perfect with a few slices of tomato on the side (100g tomato = 18 cals).

Spinach, Mushroom, Onion & Feta Flatbreads

The mere mention of 'bread' in a recipe can be intimidating, but these could not be simpler. I've chosen my favourite toppings, but of course you can vary it according to your preferences – or, indeed, what you have in the fridge.

Quantity/serves: makes 4 flatbreads

Calories per flatbread: 200

Prep time: **15 mins**

Cooking time: **15 mins**

☒ Vegan   ☑ Lacto-Ovo Vegetarian

☒ Dairy-Free   ☒ Gluten-Free

Protein 18%

Carbs 49%

Fat 33%

Ingredients

For the flatbreads
100g plain flour, plus extra for dusting
100g Greek yogurt
1 tsp baking powder
a good pinch of salt

For the topping
2 tsp neutral oil
1 small red onion, finely sliced
100g mushrooms, sliced
100g baby spinach leaves
a pinch of salt
a pinch of freshly ground black pepper
extra-virgin olive oil, for brushing
60g feta cheese
a pinch of dried chilli flakes (optional)

Method

Place the flatbread ingredients in a bowl and mix well to combine. If the mixture seems too sticky to knead, then add a bit more flour. Turn the dough out on to a well-floured surface and knead for 1 minute until it comes together in a ball. Set aside.

To make the topping, heat the oil in a frying pan over a low heat. Add the onion and fry gently until soft, then add the mushrooms. Cook for a few minutes, then turn off the heat and add in the spinach, just to wilt it down. Season well with salt and pepper.

Returning to the dough, divide it into 4 and roll into balls. Roll out each dough ball with a rolling pin to about 3mm thick, using plenty of flour to prevent sticking. Heat a large frying pan or griddle pan over a medium heat and cook the flatbreads, working 2 at a time. Cook them on one side for a few minutes until golden and starting to puff up, then flip and cook on the other side for just 1 minute. Repeat to cook the other 2 flatbreads. Use a pastry brush to brush the less-cooked side of each flatbread with extra-virgin olive oil, then spread over the vegetable mixture. Crumble over the feta and place the flatbreads under a hot grill for 1–2 minutes, until the cheese starts to melt. Sprinkle over some dried chilli flakes to serve, if you like.

Tips & Tweaks

- You can make the flatbread dough in advance, then keep it in an airtight container in the fridge for up to 3 days until you are ready to cook.
- You can spread some Rich Tomato Sauce (p. 128; 1 tbsp = 12 cals) under the toppings before you bake for more of a pizza vibe.

Shredded Brussels & Parmesan Salad

Yes, we all know that Brussels sprouts aren't just for Christmas, but it can be hard to know what else to do with them. If you think about it, they are just mini cabbages, and raw cabbage works brilliantly in salads, so why not make one with sprouts instead? A nice zingy dressing, some fresh mint and a smattering of Parmesan make this into something special.

Quantity/serves: 2

Calories per serving: 208

Prep time: **10 mins**

Cooking time: **5 mins**

☒ Vegan   ☒ Lacto-Ovo Vegetarian

☒ Dairy-Free   ☑ Gluten-Free

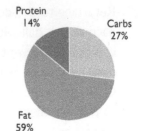

Protein 14%
Carbs 27%
Fat 59%

Ingredients

10g pine nuts
250g Brussels sprouts, outer leaves and any tough
    stalks removed, very finely sliced
a small handful of mint leaves, chopped
1 tbsp extra-virgin olive oil
½ tsp runny honey
zest and juice of ½ lemon
a pinch of salt
a pinch of freshly ground black pepper
25g Parmesan cheese, grated

Method

Place a small frying pan over a medium heat and add the pine nuts. Toast for a few minutes, tossing occasionally to brown evenly.

Place the sprouts in a serving bowl, along with the chopped mint. In a small bowl or jug, mix together the olive oil, honey, lemon juice, salt and pepper and pour this mixture over the sprouts and mint. Toss well to combine. Just before serving, top with the grated Parmesan cheese and garnish with the lemon zest and toasted pine nuts.

Tips & Tweaks

- Slicing the sprouts very thinly takes mere seconds in a food processor.
- This recipe serves 2 as a Light Day meal. To make it more substantial, top with a fried or poached egg (1 egg = 75 cals).
- On a Regular Day, this would make a lovely side dish to grilled fish or roast chicken.

Tasty Tuna Toast Topper

I have always been a fan of tuna mayo sandwiches. To this day, they probably remain my sandwich of choice, but when watching the calories, lots of bread and mayonnaise are not exactly box tickers! This is my Light Day solution.

Quantity/serves: 2

Calories per serving: 208

Prep time: 10 mins

Cooking time: 0 mins

☒ Vegan ☒ Lacto-Ovo Vegetarian

☒ Dairy-Free ☒ Gluten-Free

Protein 33%

Carbs 53%

Fat 14%

Ingredients

145g can tuna chunks in spring water, drained
1 tbsp fresh dill, finely chopped
½ red onion, finely diced
½ red pepper, finely diced
2 tbsp Greek yogurt
1 tsp lemon juice
½ tsp Dijon mustard
a pinch of salt
a pinch of freshly ground black pepper
2 slices of wholegrain bread

Method

Combine all the ingredients (except the bread!) in a bowl. Toast the bread, then top each slice with half the mixture and eat immediately.

Tips & Tweaks

- The tuna topping can be mixed up and stored in the fridge for up to 2 days.
- No butter is required on the toast – it simply adds calories, and this is tasty enough without.
- To make this even more filling, add a sliced hard-boiled egg (1 egg = 75 cals).

Beans Provençale

No matter how many recipes I create, I am always most excited by those that pack in maximum flavour for minimum effort. This one is a case in point: beans, tomatoes, some olive oil, garlic, herbs, lemon and a splash of wine. So simple, so healthy, so delicious.

Quantity/serves: 4

Calories per serving: 210

Prep time: **10 mins**

Cooking time: **45 mins**

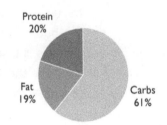

☑ Vegan (use vegan-certified wine)

☑ Lacto-Ovo Vegetarian   ☑ Dairy-Free   ☑ Gluten-Free

Ingredients

1 tbsp olive oil
1 small onion, diced
4 garlic cloves, finely grated
a few sprigs of fresh thyme, or 1 tsp dried thyme or
    dried mixed herbs
60ml dry white wine
400g can chopped tomatoes
2 × 400g cans cannellini beans, drained and rinsed
½ tsp sugar
500ml vegetable stock, made from a cube
a pinch of salt
a pinch of freshly ground pepper
zest of 1 lemon

Method

Heat the oil in a large saucepan over a medium heat. Add the onion and sauté for 3 minutes or so, then add in the garlic and thyme or dried herbs and cook for another minute. Pour the wine into the pan and swirl around. Cook for another minute, then add the tomatoes, beans, sugar and stock. Cover and reduce the heat to low. Simmer for about 30–40 minutes, stirring occasionally. You want it to reduce and thicken, but there should be some sauce left, so stop cooking when it has reduced to the right consistency. Season with salt and pepper to taste and mix through. Sprinkle over the lemon zest just before serving.

Tips & Tweaks

- You can make this in advance and keep it in the fridge for several days, or freeze.
- Snip some flat-leaf parsley over the top for a nice, fresh garnish.
- Some fresh crusty bread is ideal for soaking up the juices (1 slice = 100 cals).

Simple Veggie Tagine

A simple, veggie-packed, nourishing tagine is just the thing to fill you up for fewer calories. You can reduce the chilli powder if your family aren't spice fans, or indeed crank up the heat to your preferred level.

Quantity/serves: 4

Calories per serving: 224

Prep time: 15 mins

Cooking time: 40 mins

☑ Vegan   ☑ Lacto-Ovo Vegetarian

☑ Dairy-Free   ☑ Gluten-Free

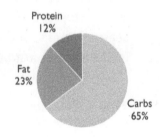

Protein 12%

Fat 23%

Carbs 65%

Ingredients

1 tbsp olive oil
1 red onion, chopped
2 garlic cloves, finely grated
2–3cm piece of fresh root ginger, finely grated
½ tsp chilli powder (or to taste)
1 tsp ground cumin
½ tsp ground turmeric
1 tsp paprika
¼ tsp ground cinnamon
10 cherry tomatoes
2 tbsp lemon juice
2 tbsp tomato purée
1kg mixed vegetables (such as aubergines, courgettes, carrots, butternut squash or peppers), cut into 2cm chunks

400g can chickpeas, drained and rinsed
a good pinch of salt
a good pinch of freshly ground black pepper

Method

Heat the oil in a large saucepan over a low heat. Add the onion and garlic and fry gently for 3–4 minutes, adding 1 tablespoon water if it gets too dry, as you don't want the mixture to go brown or stick to the pan. Add the ginger and spices and fry together for 1 minute more before adding all the remaining ingredients. Pour over enough water to just cover everything (approx. 1 litre), then season well with salt and pepper. Bring to the boil, then reduce the heat to low and cover loosely. Simmer for 40 minutes, checking and stirring occasionally. Add a little more water if it is getting too dry: you want it to retain a bit of sauce. Serve.

Tips & Tweaks

- This is a good one to make in advance and reheat – make it on a Sunday and it will improve as the week wears on.
- A spoonful of Greek yogurt stirred into this just before serving is delicious (1 tbsp = 15 cals).
- If you are doing this for the family, then it's lovely spooned over jacket potatoes – which you can have too, if it's a Regular Day (100g = 77 cals; a medium potato is about 150g).

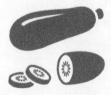

Best Black Bean Chilli

Now, it's one thing trying to eat healthily yourself, but it's a whole other thing trying to get your kids to eat your healthy creations. So, I had a 'punch the air' moment when I made this and both kids (the younger, carb-hating pescatarian and the older, carb-loving carnivore) said they LOVED it. I am resisting the urge to serve it up for every other meal in case they go off it but, suffice to say, this is a winner.

Quantity/serves: 4

Calories per serving: 230

Prep time: 10 mins

Cooking time: 40 mins

☑ Vegan   ☑ Lacto-Ovo Vegetarian

☑ Dairy-Free   ☑ Gluten-Free

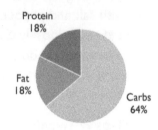

Protein 18%
Fat 18%
Carbs 64%

Ingredients

    1 tbsp olive oil
    1 small onion, finely diced
    2 tsp paprika
    2 tsp ground cumin
    2 tsp ground coriander
    ¼ tsp chilli powder (or to taste)
    2 carrots, peeled and grated
    400g can chopped tomatoes
    2 tbsp tomato purée
    1 tsp brown sugar
    a pinch of salt
    a pinch of freshly ground black pepper
    2 × 400g cans black beans, drained and rinsed

Method

Heat the oil in a large saucepan over a medium heat. Add the onion and fry gently for 3–4 minutes. Add the spices and fry for a further minute, then add the carrots and chopped tomatoes. Stir in the tomato purée and brown sugar, and add enough water to cover. Simmer for 15 minutes. If you don't want it chunky, you can blend the sauce at this point. Taste the sauce and season with the salt and pepper. Add the beans and simmer for another 20 minutes, or longer if you have time. Add a little more water if it gets too dry.

Tips & Tweaks

- If you prep the veg in advance, you can have this on the table in under half an hour.
- Serve with brown basmati rice (50g cooked weight = 65 cals) and, if you're not vegan or dairy-free, some Greek yogurt (1 tbsp = 15 cals) on the side.
- If you want to make more of a feast of it on a Regular Day, serve with grated Cheddar (if you're not vegan or dairy-free), some chopped avocado and jalapeño chillies.
- This recipe keeps brilliantly in the fridge for several days.

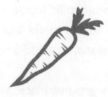

Indian Black Bean & Spinach Soup

I love black beans and I think you will too, once you've tried this soup. This is a great big bowl of goodness that will keep you going on your Light Days. It offers plenty of flavour and is extremely filling.

Quantity/serves: 2

Calories per serving: 233

Prep time: 5 mins

Cooking time: 35 mins

☑ Vegan ☑ Lacto-Ovo Vegetarian

☑ Dairy-Free ☑ Gluten-Free

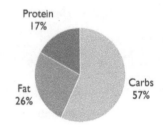

Protein 17%

Fat 26%

Carbs 57%

Ingredients

    1 tsp neutral oil
    1 small onion, diced
    2 garlic cloves, finely grated
    1 tsp mild curry powder
    1 tsp ground turmeric
    ¼ tsp chilli powder
    2 tbsp light coconut milk (optional)
    500ml vegetable stock, made from a cube
    400g can black beans, drained and rinsed
    a pinch of salt
    a pinch of freshly ground black pepper
    100g baby spinach leaves
    1 tbsp lime juice

Method

Heat the oil in a large saucepan over a low heat. Add the onion and garlic and fry until the onion softens, adding a little water if it's getting too dry. Now add the spices and mix well in the pan. Add the coconut milk (if using – see Tips & Tweaks), along with the stock and black beans, and season with salt and pepper. Simmer gently for 30 minutes. Check from time to time, and top up with a little water if it's reducing too much. Take the pan off the heat and let it cool for a few minutes, then pour the soup into a blender or food processor (or you can use a stick blender) and pulse for a few seconds: you want it to be quite chunky. Return the soup to the pan and reheat before adding the spinach and lime juice. Let the spinach wilt down, and it's ready to serve.

Tips & Tweaks

- The coconut milk is optional. It adds richness, but don't feel you have to open a tin just for this recipe. If you do, you can use the rest in one of these recipes: Brekkie in a Hurry (p. 113), Power-through Porridge with Banana, Coconut & Brown Sugar (p. 107), Simple Smoothie Bowl (p. 109), Carrot, Lemon & Ginger Soup (p. 146).
- If you're not vegan or dairy-free, try swirling in some Greek yogurt just before serving (1 tbsp = 15 cals).

Rainbow Ribbon Salad with a Tahini Dressing

Taste-wise, this salad is all about the dressing, but it looks really beautiful too. You can, for speed, grate the veggies in the food processor, but it's really not much more bother to use a hand-held vegetable peeler to create delicate ribbons – and it looks prettier, too.

Quantity/serves: 2

Calories per serving: 235

Prep time: 20 mins

Cooking time: 0 mins

☒ Vegan   ☑ Lacto-Ovo Vegetarian

☑ Dairy-Free   ☑ Gluten-Free (use tamari)

Protein 13%

Carbs 37%

Fat 50%

Ingredients

1 large carrot, peeled and shaved into ribbons
1 courgette, shaved into ribbons
½ cucumber, shaved into ribbons
1 red pepper, finely sliced

For the dressing
2 tsp soy sauce (use tamari for GF)
1 tsp honey
1 tbsp lemon juice
1 tbsp tahini
1 tbsp peanut butter or other
    nut butter
1 garlic clove, finely grated
2cm piece of fresh root ginger,
    peeled and finely grated

To garnish
20g salted peanuts, chopped
a small handful of coriander leaves (optional)

Method

Prepare the vegetables and place in a pretty bowl. Put all the
dressing ingredients in a small bowl and whisk together well to
combine. Pour the dressing over the vegetables and toss to coat.
Top with the chopped peanuts and coriander leaves and serve.

Tips & Tweaks

- You can prepare the veggies a few hours in advance and
  keep them in a bowl of cold water in the fridge, then drain,
  dry and dress just before serving.
- If you want to make this a more substantial meal, serve it
  with pan-fried fish or prawns. It goes particularly well with
  seared tuna (100g = 108 cals).

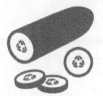

Flaky Curried Fish with Flatbreads

I think this is my family's favourite fish recipe. The curry spicing is very subtle, so it's suitable for spice-avoiders, and the soft, doughy flatbreads are just delicious. Adjust the number of flatbreads you have according to whether it's a Light Day or a Regular Day.

Quantity/serves: 4

Calories per portion (with one flatbread): 242

Prep time: **15 mins**

Cooking time: **15 mins**

☒ Vegan   ☒ Lacto-Ovo Vegetarian

☒ Dairy-Free   ☒ Gluten-Free

Protein
50%

Carbs
31%

Fat
19%

Ingredients

For the fish
1 tbsp neutral oil
2 tsp ground cumin
1 tsp mild curry powder
½ tsp ground cinnamon
½ tsp ground turmeric
a pinch of salt
a pinch of freshly ground black pepper
4 cod or haddock fillets (approx. 140g each)

For the flatbreads
200g Greek yogurt
200g chakki atta (very fine wholegrain flour) or plain
     flour, plus extra for dusting
2 tsp baking powder
¼ tsp salt

Method

Preheat the oven to 200°C/gas mark 6.

Pour the oil into a baking dish and add the spices, salt and pepper. Mix well to combine. Place the fish in the baking dish and coat with the oil and spice mixture. Set aside to marinate while you make the flatbread dough.

In a large mixing bowl, combine the flatbread ingredients with a spoon and bring together into a ball with your hands. Turn out the dough on to a well-floured surface and knead for 1–2 minutes until well combined and a little stretchy. If the mixture feels too stiff to knead, add a few drops of water.

Now place the fish in the hot oven and bake for 10–12 minutes, until the fish is moist and flakes easily. While the fish is cooking, divide the dough into 8 balls and, with your hands, flatten each ball, then use a rolling pin to roll out each one to roughly 3mm thick. Place a griddle pan or a large frying pan over a high heat, and, working in batches, cook each flatbread for 1–2 minutes on each side, until they puff up and begin to brown or have nice griddle marks on each side.

Tips & Tweaks

- You can marinate the fish and make the flatbread dough in advance, then keep in the fridge until dinner time.
- Have one flatbread on a Light Day or two on a Regular Day (1 flatbread = 100 cals).
- Roll the fish up in the flatbread with a little Greek yogurt mixed with sriracha (15 cals per tbsp) and some fresh coriander leaves.

Vietnamese-Style Chicken Salad

This recipe has been kindly donated by my good friend and fellow food writer Ghillie James, from her brilliant book *Asia Light*. It is one of my favourite mid-week salads because it is so fresh and flavour-packed, and it's really versatile in terms of what you put into it. This is my favourite combination, but you can freestyle.

Quantity/serves: 2

Calories per serving: 246

Prep time: **15 mins**

Cooking time: **2 mins**

☒ Vegan   ☒ Lacto-Ovo Vegetarian

☑ Dairy-Free   ☑ Gluten-Free

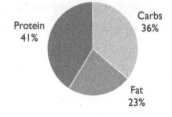

Protein 41%

Carbs 36%

Fat 23%

Ingredients

1 tsp sesame seeds
75g green beans, trimmed and halved
1 celery stick, sliced
½ red or yellow pepper, sliced
100g bean sprouts
¼ cucumber, diced
200g cooked chicken, no skin, shredded
2 spring onions, sliced
a small handful of fresh mint leaves, chopped

For the dressing
1 tbsp fish sauce (*nam pla*)
1 tsp rice vinegar (or other white vinegar)
1 tbsp runny honey
1 small red chilli, deseeded and chopped

1 garlic clove, finely grated
juice of 1 lime
1 tsp sesame oil

Method

Heat a small frying pan over a medium heat. Add the sesame seeds and toast for 1 minute, then set aside in a small bowl. Return the pan to the hob to make the dressing, this time over a low heat. Add the fish sauce, rice vinegar, honey, chilli, garlic and lime juice to the pan and bring to a simmer. Stir for a further minute or so, then turn off the heat. Stir in the sesame oil and set aside to cool.

Bring a small saucepan of water to the boil. Add the green beans and blanch for 1 minute. Drain and run under the cold tap so they retain their nice green colour, then transfer to a serving bowl. Add the celery, pepper, bean sprouts and cucumber and toss together. Top with the shredded chicken, spring onions and mint leaves. Pour over the dressing just before serving, and top with the toasted sesame seeds.

Tips & Tweaks

- You can make the dressing and get all the other ingredients prepped and chopped in the fridge in advance – then it's just an assembly job.
- You need cooked chicken for this, so if you don't have leftovers, buy a pre-cooked breast and remove the skin.

Italian Aubergines

I am an absolute sucker for aubergine Parmigiana, so creating this lighter version was a challenge I was very happy to take on. It uses the Rich Tomato Sauce on p. 128, so be sure to have some on hand. Otherwise, it's a cinch to make.

Quantity/serves: 4

Calories per serving: 258

Prep time: **10 mins**

Cooking time: **50 mins**

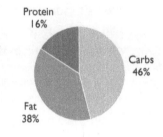

Protein 16%

Carbs 46%

Fat 38%

☒ Vegan   ☒ Lacto-Ovo Vegetarian

☒ Dairy-Free   ☑ Gluten-Free

Ingredients

> 1kg aubergines (approx. 2 large aubergines), topped, tailed and cut lengthways into 1–1.5cm thick slices
> 1 tbsp olive oil, plus extra for greasing
> 200g cherry tomatoes
> 500g Rich Tomato Sauce (p. 128)
> a handful of basil leaves
> 120g ricotta cheese
> 30g Parmesan cheese, grated
> a pinch of freshly ground black pepper

Method

Preheat the oven to 180°C/gas mark 4 and lightly grease a baking tray with olive oil.

Place the aubergine slices on the baking tray and lightly brush with the olive oil. Place in the oven for 20 minutes. After 20 minutes, remove from the oven and gently turn over the aubergine slices. Scatter over the cherry tomatoes and return to the oven for 10 more minutes.

Take a 25 × 20cm baking dish, and brush the base with some of the Rich Tomato Sauce. Place a layer of cooked aubergine slices over the sauce, then add some of the cherry tomatoes and place a couple of basil leaves on each slice. Dot with ricotta, then cover everything with a thin layer of tomato sauce. Repeat this process in layers until all the ingredients have been used up, finishing with a layer of tomato sauce. Sprinkle over the grated Parmesan and a pinch of black pepper, then return to the oven for 20 minutes until the cheese has melted and turned golden.

Tips & Tweaks

- If using pre-made, frozen Rich Tomato Sauce, remove it from the freezer in the morning so it has enough time to defrost.
- You can assemble this earlier in the day, ready to bake at dinner time.
- If you're making this for the family and they don't all like aubergine, you could do half using some wholewheat lasagne sheets (parboil first), and the other half with aubergine.
- On a Regular Day, you can double the amount of Parmesan on top and have a nice slice of sourdough bread to mop up the sauce – this adds 130 cals per serving.

Hearty Veggie Soba Miso Soup

This is an absolute go-to recipe in my house: we all love Japanese food, and it's simple, healthy and tasty. If you haven't tried soba noodles before, they are delicious. Made from buckwheat, they have a slightly nutty flavour and work beautifully with the umami of the miso.

Quantity/serves: 2

Calories per serving: 260

Prep time: **10 mins**

Cooking time: **15 mins**

☑ Vegan   ☑ Lacto-Ovo Vegetarian

☑ Dairy-Free

☑ Gluten-Free (make sure soba noodles are 100% buckwheat)

Protein
11%

Fat
31%

Carbs
58%

Ingredients

1 tsp sesame seeds, toasted (optional)
60g dried soba noodles
2 tsp sesame oil
1 tsp neutral oil
1 garlic clove, finely grated
2cm piece of fresh root ginger, peeled and finely grated
100g leeks, finely sliced
2 tbsp miso paste
½ small carrot, peeled and grated
100g baby spinach leaves
2 spring onions, sliced
1 small green chilli, deseeded and finely sliced
    (optional)

Method

If you are planning to garnish with sesame seeds, toast them in a dry frying pan over a medium heat until they turn golden, then set aside.

Half-fill a medium-sized saucepan with water and place it over a medium heat. Bring to the boil, then add the soba noodles and simmer for 4 minutes. Drain and place in a bowl. Add the sesame oil and toss to coat, then set aside until needed.

Return the same saucepan to a low–medium heat and add the neutral oil. Add the garlic and ginger and gently fry for 1 minute, then add the leeks. If it's all getting a bit dry, add a couple of tablespoons of water. Let the leeks soften for a couple of minutes. In the meantime, pour 500ml boiling water into a measuring jug and add the miso paste. Whisk with a fork until fully dissolved, then add to the saucepan. Bring to the boil, then add the carrot and spinach leaves. Let it cook for 30 seconds.

Divide the noodles between 2 serving bowls before pouring the soup over each. Garnish with the spring onions and chilli and serve.

Tips & Tweaks

- Prep all the veggies and weigh out the noodles before you start – once you get going, it all happens quite quickly.
- Eat this soup straight away while the veggies are still fresh and crunchy.
- This is suitable for a Light Day (30g noodles per serving). On a Regular Day, you can double the noodles to 60g per serving (adds 100 cals per serving).
- To make a more substantial meal, add some cooked prawns (75g = 60 cals).

Pot Noodles

Noodles are definitely a fallback lunch that everyone seems to love. This recipe is endlessly flexible, so use it to finish up whatever veggies you have in the fridge.

Quantity/serves: 1

Calories per serving: 260

Prep time: 15 mins

Cooking time: 10 mins

☒ Vegan (see Tips & Tweaks)

☒ Lacto-Ovo Vegetarian (see Tips & Tweaks)

☑ Dairy-Free ☒ Gluten-Free (see Tips & Tweaks)

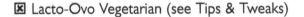

Protein 25%

Carbs 60%

Fat 15%

Ingredients

40g dried vermicelli rice noodles, broken up
50g thinly sliced or grated mixed vegetables (such as spring onion, carrot, red pepper or courgette)
25g green leaves (such as spinach, pak choi or chard), roughly chopped
50g cooked prawns or chicken
½ tsp sesame oil
2 tsp soy sauce
1 tsp lime juice
½ red chilli, finely chopped
2cm piece of fresh root ginger, peeled and finely grated
300ml hot vegetable stock, made from a cube
a few coriander leaves (optional)

Method

Use a large heatproof jar with a lid if you have one; if not, use a medium heatproof bowl. Place the noodles, vegetables and prawns or chicken in the bottom of the jar or bowl. In a small bowl or jug, mix together the sesame oil, soy sauce, lime juice, ginger and chilli, then tip into the jar/bowl. When you're ready to eat, pour over the hot stock, then cover with a lid or a piece of cling film and leave to soak for 10 minutes. Serve, with a few coriander leaves on top if you like.

Tips & Tweaks

- This is a great lunch to take to work, as long as you have access to a kettle. Just take it with you in a jar, and when you're ready to eat, crumble over half a stock cube before topping up with boiling water and mixing well.
- For a vegan version, replace the prawns and chicken with tofu.
- To make this gluten-free, just swap the soy sauce for tamari.
- On a Regular Day, top with a quartered hard-boiled egg for extra protein (1 egg = 75 cals).

Teriyaki Mackerel with Sesame Spinach

If mackerel isn't something you eat on a regular basis, then it really should be: it's a super healthy oily fish, it's sustainable and it's cheap. Keep some fillets in the freezer for this quick, family-friendly supper.

Quantity/serves: 4

Calories per serving: 267

Prep time: 5 mins

Cooking time: 20 mins

☒ Vegan ☒ Lacto-Ovo Vegetarian

☑ Dairy-Free ☒ Gluten-Free (see Tips & Tweaks)

Protein
33%

Carbs
10%

Fat
57%

Ingredients

4 fresh mackerel fillets (approx. 100g each)

For the teriyaki marinade
3 tbsp soy sauce
2 tbsp rice wine vinegar
1 tbsp honey
1 garlic clove, finely sliced
3cm piece of fresh root ginger,
    cut into matchsticks

For the sesame spinach
1 tsp sesame seeds
2 tsp sesame oil
200g spinach leaves
a pinch of salt
a pinch of freshly ground black pepper

Method

Preheat the oven to 200°C/gas mark 6.

In a small bowl or jug, mix together all the marinade ingredients, then pour into a baking dish. Add the mackerel fillets, toss them in the marinade and then arrange them in a row, skin-side up. Cover with tin foil and place in the hot oven for 15 minutes.

Meanwhile, toast the sesame seeds in a dry frying pan over a medium heat for 2–3 minutes until golden. Set aside.

Place a large frying pan or wok over a medium heat and add the sesame oil. When the oil is hot, add the spinach leaves and season with salt and pepper. Stir gently for a minute or so while the spinach wilts. Turn off the heat and let it continue wilting for another minute or so. Place in a serving bowl and sprinkle over the toasted sesame seeds.

When the mackerel is ready, remove from the oven and preheat the grill to high. Take off the foil and place the fish under the hot grill for 5 minutes or so for the skin to crisp up. Serve immediately, with the spinach on the side.

Tips & Tweaks

- You can prep the fish in advance and leave it to marinate for 2 hours in the fridge: it will taste even better.
- To make this gluten-free, just swap the soy sauce for tamari.
- On a Regular Day, serve with brown rice (100g cooked weight = 110 cals).

Warm Spinach Salad with Feta & Strawberries

I ate a version of this one Sunday at a little café near where I live, and it was so delicious I had to try and recreate it. I love the hot and cold elements of this dish, and strawberries and feta make a delicious combination.

Quantity/serves: 2

Calories per serving: 277

Prep time: 15 mins

Cooking time: 5 mins

☒ Vegan   ☑ Lacto-Ovo Vegetarian

☒ Dairy-Free   ☑ Gluten-Free

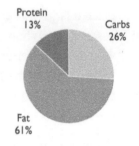

Protein 13%
Carbs 26%
Fat 61%

Ingredients

20g pine nuts
100g sugar snap peas
100g broccoli florets
½ red onion, sliced
1 tbsp extra-virgin olive oil
1 tbsp red wine vinegar
1 tsp honey
50g feta cheese, chopped into 1cm cubes
a pinch of freshly ground black pepper
100g baby spinach leaves
50g strawberries, sliced

Method

Heat a small frying pan over a medium heat and toast the pine nuts for 1–2 minutes until golden. Place in a bowl and set aside.

Heat a large frying pan or wok over a low heat. Add 2 tablespoons water, followed by the sugar snap peas, broccoli and red onion. Cover with a lid and steam for 5 minutes. Remove the vegetables from the pan and place them in a large salad bowl. Take the pan off the heat and add the oil, vinegar and honey to it to make a dressing. Mix together and pour over the vegetables. Add the cubed feta to the salad bowl, along with a good grind of black pepper and mix well. Now add the spinach leaves and strawberries and toss lightly. Sprinkle over the toasted pine nuts to serve.

Tips & Tweaks

- This is best eaten straight away while the veggies are warm.
- If you don't have strawberries, ripe peach slices would work equally well.
- Add some cooked chicken (100g = 165 cals) if you want to make it a bit more substantial on a Regular Day.

Fast Fish Pie

This recipe has kindly been shared with me by Mimi Spencer from her fantastic book *Fast Cook*, an absolute treasure trove of delicious, low-calorie meals. The masterstroke here is using filo instead of mashed potato to keep the calorie count where it needs to be on a Light Day.

Quantity/serves: 4

Calories per serving: 278

Prep time: **10 mins**

Cooking time: **35 mins**

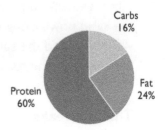

☒ Vegan   ☒ Lacto-Ovo Vegetarian

☒ Dairy-Free   ☒ Gluten-Free

Ingredients

spray oil
250g bag of spinach leaves
200g half-fat crème fraîche
a handful of fresh dill, chopped
a handful of fresh flat-leaf parsley, chopped
1 tbsp Dijon mustard
1 tsp lemon juice
250g skinless white fish fillets, cut into chunks
250g skinless smoked haddock fillets, cut into chunks
300g cooked king prawns
a pinch of salt
a pinch of freshly ground black pepper
3–4 sheets filo pastry

Method

Preheat the oven to 180°C/gas mark 4 and lightly spray an ovenproof dish with oil.

Pierce the bag of spinach and microwave on full power for 90 seconds. If you don't have a microwave, wilt the spinach in a large frying pan over a low heat. Once the spinach has wilted, squeeze out as much moisture as possible by pressing it firmly between sheets of kitchen roll. Cover the base of the ovenproof dish with the spinach.

In a bowl, mix together the crème fraîche, dill, parsley, mustard, lemon juice, fish and prawns. Season with salt and pepper and spoon this mixture over the layer of spinach. Spray the filo sheets with a little oil, then scrunch them up and place on top of the fish mix. Bake for 25–30 minutes until the filo is crisp.

Tips & Tweaks

- Add a couple of halved, hard-boiled eggs to the pie for some extra protein (1 egg = 75 cals).
- This goes really well with some blanched green beans on the side (100g serving = 31 cals).
- To make this more substantial for the rest of the family, serve with some mashed potato. If it's a Regular Day, you can add some to your plate, too.

Black Bean Fritters with Avocado Dip

Black beans are fantastic because, being packed with fibre, they are super filling. They are also the one bean my kids actually like rather than just tolerate, so you'll find them in a few recipes in this book: try the Best Black Bean Chilli on p. 166 or, for a healthy treat, the Black Bean Brownies on p. 236 are a revelation.

Quantity/serves: 4

Calories per serving: 286

Prep time: 15 mins

Cooking time: 25 mins

☒ Vegan   ☑ Lacto-Ovo Vegetarian

☒ Dairy-Free   ☑ Gluten-Free

Protein 18%

Carbs 48%

Fat 34%

Ingredients

For the fritters
2 tsp neutral oil
1 small red onion, finely diced
2 garlic cloves, finely grated
2 tsp ground cumin
¼ tsp cayenne pepper (or to taste)
2 × 400g cans black beans, drained and rinsed
2 heaped tbsp ground almonds, plus extra to coat
a pinch of salt
a pinch of freshly ground black pepper

For the dip
1 avocado, peeled, stoned and mashed
100ml Greek yogurt
1 garlic clove, finely grated

1 tomato, diced
juice of 1 lime

Method

Heat 1 teaspoon of the oil in a large frying pan over a low heat.
Add the onions and garlic and sauté for 2–3 minutes until softened.
Add the spices and continue to fry for another minute or so, then
transfer the mixture to a food processor, along with half the black
beans. Pulse the mixture to a coarse paste, then transfer to a bowl.
Add the ground almonds, the rest of the black beans, and the salt
and pepper and combine well. Form into 12 equally sized fritters
and coat lightly with more ground almonds. Using the same frying
pan, heat the remaining oil over a medium heat. Fry the fritters for
5 minutes on each side until golden; you will probably have to work
in two batches.

To make the dip, mix together the mashed avocado and yogurt in
a bowl until well combined, then stir in the garlic, tomato and lime
juice. Keep in the fridge until ready to serve.

Tips & Tweaks

- The fritters can be prepared in advance and kept in the
  fridge until you're ready to cook, or frozen.
- I serve these with a simple salad of grated carrot dressed
  with apple cider vinegar or red wine vinegar (100g =
  42 cals).

Tagliata & Watercress with a Mustard Orange Dressing

Tagliata is a rather lovely Italian word for sliced-up steak, usually served quite pink and on a bed of peppery leaves with some Parmesan shavings. I've put my twist on it with an orange and mustard dressing, which adds a little bit of sweetness and tang. Such a simple dish, but always extremely popular in our house.

Quantity/serves: 4

Calories per serving: 289

Prep time: 10 mins

Cooking time: 10 mins

☒ Vegan   ☒ Lacto-Ovo Vegetarian

☒ Dairy-Free   ☑ Gluten-Free

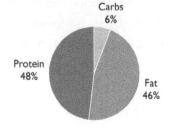

Carbs 6%

Protein 48%

Fat 46%

Ingredients

200g watercress

30g walnuts, chopped

400g sirloin steak (approx. 2cm thick), any excess fat trimmed

1 tsp olive oil

a pinch of salt

a pinch of freshly ground black pepper

30g Parmesan cheese, peeled into fine shavings

For the dressing

1 tbsp extra-virgin olive oil

juice of 1 orange

2 tsp Dijon mustard

2 tsp apple cider vinegar

a pinch of salt
a pinch of freshly ground black pepper

Method

Arrange the watercress on a serving plate and set aside. In a small bowl or jug, mix together all the dressing ingredients and set aside.

Place a small frying pan over a medium heat. Add the chopped walnuts and toast for 1–2 minutes until starting to brown, then transfer to a bowl and set aside.

Now you are ready to fry the steak, which won't take long. Rub the steak all over with the olive oil and season well with salt and pepper. Place a large, non-stick frying pan over a high heat. Once the pan is really hot, add the steak. Cook for 2 minutes on each side for medium–rare or 3 minutes for medium, turning it only once so you get a nice browning on each side. Set the steak aside on a plate to rest for 2 minutes, then carve into thick slices using a sharp knife.

To serve, pour some of the dressing over the watercress and sprinkle over the toasted nuts and Parmesan shavings. Place the steak slices on top and pour over any juices that have come out of the meat while it has been resting. Serve with the rest of the dressing in a jug on the side.

Tips & Tweaks

- Make sure the steak is at room temperature before cooking. You need to take it out of the fridge an hour or so beforehand.
- Use a vegetable peeler to shave the Parmesan into curls.
- I like to serve this with baked hasselback potatoes: just carefully slice across the width of the potatoes at about 2mm intervals, rub with olive oil, season and bake for 1 hour at 180°C/gas mark 4 (1 medium-sized hasselback potato, approx. 150g = 135 calories).

Baked Sweet Potatoes with Tzatziki

If ever there was a match made in heaven, this is surely it: starchy sweet potatoes and creamy, tangy tzatziki – to echo that much overused phrase, what's not to love? If you keep an eye on the portion size, there's no reason why you can't have a hit of carbs on a Light Day.

Quantity/serves: 2

Calories per serving: 299

Prep time: 10 mins

Cooking time: **45–60 mins**

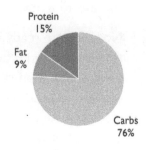

☒ Vegan   ☑ Lacto-Ovo Vegetarian

☒ Dairy-Free   ☑ Gluten-Free

Ingredients

2 small sweet potatoes (approx. 500g total), scrubbed
150ml Greek yogurt
100g cucumber, grated
1 garlic clove, finely grated
1 tsp extra-virgin olive oil
1 tsp white vinegar (or use another clear vinegar, such as apple cider or white wine, etc.)
1 tbsp finely chopped fresh dill
a pinch of salt

Method

Preheat the oven to 200°C/gas mark 6. Place the sweet potatoes on a baking tray and place in the oven. Bake for 45 minutes–1 hour, depending on the size of the sweet potatoes. When they're ready, they should be tender when pierced with a knife.

Meanwhile, make the tzatziki. Wrap the grated cucumber in some kitchen roll, and squeeze to take out most of the liquid. Place the cucumber in a bowl and add the garlic, Greek yogurt, olive oil, vinegar, dill and salt. Mix well to combine, then transfer to the fridge until the potatoes are ready.

Remove the potatoes from the oven. Place each one on a plate and cut in half. Drizzle the cut sides with the tzatziki (using half for each potato) and serve.

Tips & Tweaks

- The tzatziki can easily be made up the day before: in fact, it tastes even better if you do.
- If the kids aren't sweet potato fans, just make regular baked potatoes for them: the tzatziki goes well with them, too.
- On a Regular Day, have this as a side dish with some seared pork medallions (100g serving = 135 cals).

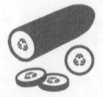

Salmon & Prawn Chowder

Chowder is a strange word, isn't it? I've looked it up so you don't have to, and apparently it's a corruption of the French word *chaudière*, or cauldron. So there you go. I don't make this in a cauldron, by the way, but it still tastes absolutely delicious.

Quantity/serves: 2

Calories per serving: 299

Prep time: **15 mins**

Cooking time: **30 mins**

☒ Vegan   ☒ Lacto-Ovo Vegetarian

☒ Dairy-Free   ☒ Gluten-Free

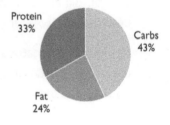

Protein 33%

Carbs 43%

Fat 24%

Ingredients

250ml semi-skimmed milk
1 salmon fillet (approx. 100g)
50g raw tiger prawns, halved lengthways
1 tsp olive oil
½ onion, finely chopped
¼ leek, finely sliced
1 tsp plain flour
1 potato (approx. 100g), chopped into 1cm dice
25g dried red lentils
500ml fish or vegetable stock, made from a cube
1 tsp Dijon mustard
a pinch of salt
a pinch of freshly ground black pepper
a small handful of fresh flat-leaf parsley, chopped

Method

Gently heat the milk in a small saucepan over a low heat. Add the fish and prawns to the hot milk and poach for 5 minutes, being careful not to let the milk boil. Remove the fish and prawns with a slotted spoon and set aside on a plate to cool. Set aside the milk, too, to add back in later.

Place a medium-sized saucepan pan over a medium heat and add the oil, onion and leek. Sauté for 3–4 minutes, then add the flour, potato and lentils and mix well. Stir in the stock and mustard, then leave to simmer gently for 15 minutes. Add the reserved milk and heat through, then taste and season. Remove the salmon skin and flake the flesh, then add this to the soup along with the prawns. Sprinkle over the parsley and serve.

Tips & Tweaks

- Serve with lemon wedges on the side to squeeze over.
- Have a bowl on its own on a Light Day, or with a piece of bread on a Regular Day (1 slice = 100 cals).

Quick Lunch Assemblies

Lunch is often a grab 'n' go affair, and while there are loads of lovely lunch recipes in this book, including time-saving soups you can make in advance, you will have the odd day where you haven't had time to think ahead and just need something quick, healthy and low-cal to hand. Here are some ideas:

Chicken & Hummus Romaine Wraps

Serves: 1

Calories per serving: 117

Fat: 28%   Protein: 37%   Carbs: 35%

Ingredients

> 2 large romaine (or iceberg) lettuce leaves
> 2 tbsp hummus or Coronation Hummus (p. 126)
> 2 slices of cold, cooked chicken (approx. 50g)
> a few slices of chopped cucumber, red pepper,
>   shredded carrot – whatever you have in the fridge

Method

Spread each lettuce leaf with 1 tablespoon hummus. Top with a slice of chicken, add the veggies and roll up to make two wraps. Use a cocktail stick to secure if the lettuce keeps flapping open.

Avocado on Toast with Spicy Seeds

Serves: 1

Calories per serving: 272

Fat: 50%   Protein: 16%   Carbs: 34%

Ingredients

1 slice of wholegrain bread
¼ ripe avocado
25g feta cheese
1 tsp Spicy Seeds Topper (p. 122)

Method

I strongly urge you to make up some of my Spicy Seeds Topper, as it is such a flavour saviour on a busy day. Toast the bread, squish on the avocado, crumble over the feta and sprinkle the seeds over the top.

Quick Chickpea Salad

Serves: 2

Calories per serving: 210

Fat: 24%   Protein: 16%   Carbs: 60%

Ingredients

400g can chickpeas, drained and rinsed
½ red pepper, diced
¼ cucumber, diced
1 tsp extra-virgin olive oil
1 tsp red wine vinegar
a pinch of salt
a pinch of paprika

Method

Place all the ingredients in a bowl and toss well. This keeps well in the fridge, so it can make two Light Day lunches or a nice side dish on a Regular Day.

Some other Quick Lunch Assemblies under 300 calories:

- **Tuna & Bean Salad** – Mix together ½ 400g can white beans, ½ 145g can tuna (in spring water), sliced red onion and plenty of chopped salad veg (such as cucumber, peppers, carrots). Dress with 1 tsp olive oil and a squeeze of lemon juice. Serve with a couple of crispbread crackers.

- **Curried Egg Open Sandwich** – Place some cucumber slices on 1 slice of wholegrain bread. Top with 1 hard-boiled egg mixed with 1 tsp mayonnaise, a good pinch of curry powder, and salt and pepper. No butter needed.

- **Sardines on Toast** – Squash a 120g can of good old-fashioned sardines in tomato sauce on to 1 slice of wholegrain toast, and dust with plenty of black pepper.

- **Greek Salad Wholemeal Pitta** – Mix together some chopped red pepper, cucumber, cherry tomatoes and olives with a little sliced red onion and crumbled feta. Dress with some red wine vinegar and stuff into a split wholemeal pitta bread.

- **Tomatoes on Sourdough Toast** – Rub 1 raw garlic clove over 1 slice of sourdough toast, then pile on some sliced ripe tomatoes. Top with torn basil leaves, a drizzle of balsamic vinegar and a little salt and black pepper.

- **Quick Spinach Omelette Wrap** – Wilt a handful of spinach leaves in a pan, then add two whisked eggs and cook to make a thin omelette, adding a pinch of dried chilli flakes if you like. Use the omelette as a wrap for any veggies you have in the fridge (tomatoes, spring onions, grated carrot, etc.).

- **Vegetable Stir-fry with an Egg** – Fry some sliced onion and garlic in a pan with a little olive oil. Chop up a selection of veg (such as broccoli, beans, asparagus, mushrooms and peppers) and add to the pan. Cook until softened, then season well and put on a plate. Fry an egg in the same pan, pop it on top of the veggies and grate over a little Parmesan cheese to serve.

- **Prawn Avo Salad** – Combine 75g cooked prawns with ½ chopped avocado, salad leaves, chopped cucumber and any chopped fresh herbs you might have left in the salad drawer. Dress with a simple oil and vinegar vinaigrette.

- **Quick Tabbouleh** – Place about 30g bulgur wheat (or wholegrain couscous) in a bowl, cover with boiling water and let stand for 10 mins or until softened. Meanwhile, finely chop a large handful of parsley and mint leaves and some tomato and onion. Dress with 1 tsp olive oil and 1 tsp lemon juice and season well. Fluff up the bulgur or couscous with a fork and add to the other ingredients. Combine well and serve.

- **Cottage Cheese with Olive Oil & Black Pepper** – Put 150g cottage cheese in a bowl and season with salt and pepper. If you like, add some chopped tomato, spring onion, chives or other fresh herbs. Drizzle over a little extra-virgin olive oil and enjoy with some oatcakes or wholegrain crackers.

Paprika Roast Cauli & Sweet Potatoes
with Feta

Roasted cauliflower is definitely a 'thing' right now, and about time, too! For far too long, cauliflower was an unloved veg, destined to be boiled and bland. Not so here: tossed in spices and roasted with sweet potatoes, onions and seasoned with feta, this packs a huge, healthy flavour punch.

Quantity/serves: 2

Calories per serving: 308

Prep time: 10 mins

Cooking time: 35 mins

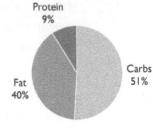

☒ Vegan ☑ Lacto-Ovo Vegetarian

☒ Dairy-Free ☑ Gluten-Free

Ingredients

1 tbsp olive oil
1 tsp paprika
1 tsp ground cumin
1 tsp ground coriander
2 garlic cloves, peeled and finely grated
3cm piece of fresh root ginger, peeled and finely grated
400g cauliflower florets
200g sweet potatoes, peeled and cubed
1 large red onion, peeled and cut into chunks
a good pinch of salt
a good pinch of freshly ground black pepper
10g pine nuts
25g feta cheese

Method

Preheat the oven to 180°C/gas mark 4.

In a large bowl, mix together the oil, paprika, cumin, coriander, garlic and ginger. Add the cauliflower, sweet potatoes and red onion and toss in the spice mix to coat well, then spread the vegetables evenly over the base of a roasting tin. Sprinkle over the salt and pepper and place in the oven. After 20 minutes, remove the tin from the oven and mix everything up really well, then return to the oven for a further 15 minutes. In the meantime, toast the pine nuts in a hot frying pan over a medium heat until golden. When the vegetables are done, remove from the oven and place on a serving plate. Sprinkle over the toasted pine nuts and crumble over the feta cheese, then serve.

Tips & Tweaks

- This makes a great lunch on a Light Day, or make a double quantity so that you can have some as a side dish on a Regular Day, too.
- Mix this with bulgur wheat on a Regular Day to make a more substantial meal (100g cooked weight = 84 cals).
- Scatter over some chopped flat-leaf parsley for extra freshness.

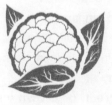

Aubergine, Lentil, Red Pepper & Olive Stew

I channelled my inner Ottolenghi (yes, him again!) for this one — indeed, he does something similar with tomatoes instead of peppers, but the combination of peppers and aubergines somehow makes the whole thing a bit more substantial. As you may have noticed, I love things that can be made in advance and then heated up over the course of a few days to make easy low-cal meals a breeze. This is no exception.

Quantity/serves: 4

Calories per serving: 313

Prep time: **15 mins**

Cooking time: **45 mins**

☑ Vegan (use certified vegan wine)

☑ Lacto-Ovo Vegetarian   ☑ Dairy-Free   ☑ Gluten-Free

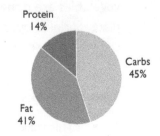

Protein 14%

Carbs 45%

Fat 41%

Ingredients

3 tbsp olive oil
1 red onion, finely diced
3 garlic cloves, finely sliced
2 tsp dried mixed herbs
1 tsp ground cinnamon
a pinch of dried chilli flakes (to taste)
200g aubergine, cut into chunks
1 red pepper, sliced
150g dried green or brown lentils
500ml vegetable stock, made from a cube
50ml dry white wine
a pinch of salt
a pinch of freshly ground black pepper

100g whole green olives, with stones
a small handful of flat-leaf parsley, chopped

Method

Heat 2 tablespoons of the oil in a large saucepan over a low heat.
Add the onion, garlic, mixed herbs, cinnamon and chilli flakes, and
gently sauté for 5 minutes. Remove the mixture from the pan and
set aside in a bowl. Add the remaining oil to the pan, followed by
the aubergine and red pepper. Sauté for 10 minutes, until the skins
of the vegetables are starting to brown. Return the onion mixture
to the pan, along with the lentils, stock and wine, and simmer gently
for 20 minutes. Check the seasoning and add salt and pepper as
required. If the stew is getting too dry, you can add 100ml water.
Stir in the olives and simmer for a further 10 minutes until the
lentils are tender. Scatter over the flat-leaf parsley to serve.

Tips & Tweaks

- This keeps very well in the fridge: a good one for Sunday
  meal prep.
- Scoop this up with a wholemeal pitta bread (1 pitta bread =
  145 cals).
- Some Greek yogurt swirled in just before serving tastes
  lovely (1 tbsp = 15 cals).

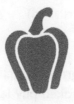

Puy Lentil & Tomato Salad with Goat's Cheese & Green Chilli

So, you know when you rashly offer to bring something round to a friend's house for lunch and then realise you haven't got anything in? No? Just me then! Well, this salad was the result of such a situation. I happened to have some pouches of pre-cooked puy lentils, some cherry tomatoes and some goat's cheese and the rest, as they say, is . . . well, not exactly history, but it *is* a very delicious salad or side dish.

Quantity/serves: 2

Calories per serving: 315

Prep time: 15 mins

Cooking time: 0 mins

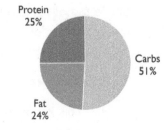

Protein 25%

Carbs 51%

Fat 24%

☒ Vegan   ☑ Lacto-Ovo Vegetarian

☒ Dairy-Free   ☑ Gluten-Free

Ingredients

2 tbsp Greek yogurt
50g soft goat's cheese
1 small green chilli, deseeded and finely chopped
¼ tsp ground cardamom (or seeds from 2–3 pods, removed and crushed)
juice of 1 lime
a pinch of salt
a pinch of freshly ground black pepper
250g pouch pre-cooked puy lentils
10 cherry tomatoes, halved
½ small red onion, finely sliced

1 tsp extra-virgin olive oil
a few mint leaves, chopped

Method

Place the yogurt, goat's cheese, chilli, cardamom, half the lime juice and the salt and pepper in a blender and whizz up to make a creamy dressing. Place the puy lentils in a serving bowl and break up with a fork if they are a bit stuck together. Add the dressing and mix well to combine. In a separate bowl, toss the tomatoes and onion in the olive oil and remaining lime juice, then place this mixture on top of the dressed lentils. Add the chopped mint leaves to garnish and serve.

Tips & Tweaks

- As this salad is leaf-free, you can make it in advance and stash it in the fridge – add the mint garnish just before serving.
- This is a lovely side dish for a barbecue, as it complements grilled food really well.

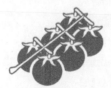

Quickest Ever Spinach & Chickpea Curry

I have to admit to an almost obsessive need to create recipes that pack the biggest flavour punch for the least effort, and I think I've cracked it with this one. When I put this on Instagram, it was one of my most popular posts, so it looks like there are a lot of people out there who are of the same mind.

Quantity/serves: 2

Calories per serving: 323

Prep time: **10 mins**

Cooking time: **30 mins**

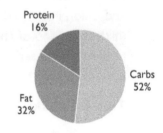

☑ Vegan   ☑ Lacto-Ovo Vegetarian

☑ Dairy-Free   ☑ Gluten-Free

Ingredients

    1 tbsp neutral oil
    1 red onion, finely sliced
    1 garlic clove, finely grated
    1 tsp ground cumin
    1 tsp ground coriander
    1 tsp ground turmeric
    ½ tsp cayenne pepper or hot chilli powder
        (or more to taste)
    400g can chickpeas, drained and rinsed
    400g can chopped tomatoes
    1 vegetable stock cube
    juice of ½ lemon
    a good pinch of salt
    a good pinch of black pepper
    a couple of big handfuls of spinach leaves, rinsed

Method

Heat the oil in a large saucepan over a low heat. Add the onion and garlic and sauté gently for a couple of minutes until they have softened. Add all the spices and stir for a further 30 seconds before adding the chickpeas and tomatoes. Stir well, then crumble in the stock cube. Add the lemon juice, along with 200ml water, and season well with salt and pepper. Simmer gently for around 25 minutes. If it looks to be reducing too much, add a little more water. Stir in the spinach, let it wilt for a minute or two, and it's ready to eat.

Tips & Tweaks

- This tastes even better the next day, so make a double batch on a Sunday and you've got a couple of quick and easy meals in the bag already.
- Stir in a blob of Greek yogurt (1 tbsp = 15 cals) just before serving for extra zing.
- Pair with a homemade flatbread (p. 156; 1 flatbread = 100 cals) on a Regular Day.

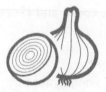

Harissa-spiced Pork Tenderloin with Roast Apples

It's always a good idea to have something a bit fancy you can get together for, well, a get together, and this one fits the bill nicely. If you get the pork marinating early, you'll be rewarded with better flavour later on. The bonus with pork tenderloin is the quick cooking time, which, happily enough, is about the same amount of time it takes to roast the apples.

Quantity/serves: 4

Calories per serving: 336

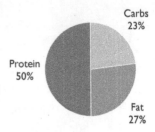

Prep time: 10 mins (plus marinating time)

Cooking time: 25–30 mins

☒ Vegan ☒ Lacto-Ovo Vegetarian

☑ Dairy-Free ☑ Gluten-Free

Ingredients

2 pork tenderloins (approx. 300g each)
2 large apples, cored and sliced, skin on
1 tsp olive oil

For the marinade
1 garlic clove, finely grated
1 tbsp extra-virgin olive oil
juice of ½ lemon
1 tbsp harissa
1 tbsp date syrup or black treacle
1 tsp ground cinnamon
1 tsp ground cumin
1 tsp paprika

a pinch of salt
a pinch of freshly ground black pepper

Method

Mix together all the marinade ingredients in a bowl. Coat the pork tenderloins in the marinade and leave to marinate (see Tips & Tweaks).

When it's time to cook, preheat the oven to 200°C/gas mark 6.

Coat the apples with the olive oil and place them around the outside of a roasting tin. Take the thin ends of the marinated tenderloins and fold them over, securing them with a cocktail stick: this prevents the ends cooking too quickly and becoming overdone. Heat a large frying pan over a high heat and sear the tenderloins for around 1 minute on each side. Now place the pork in the roasting tin with the apples and roast in the oven for 20 minutes – if you have a meat thermometer, you are looking for an internal reading of 65°C.

Once cooked, remove the meat from the tin and allow to rest under some tin foil for 10 minutes. Pour any roasting juices into a jug for serving with the meat. You can switch off the oven and leave the apples inside to keep warm while the meat is resting. Remember to pour any juices that are released from the meat while it's resting into the jug along with the roasting juices. When it's time to serve, slice the pork and arrange on a serving plate with the apples, with the jug of juices on the side.

Tips & Tweaks

- The pork ideally needs to marinate for at least 3 hours in the fridge. Take it out 1 hour before cooking so the meat comes up to room temperature.
- The roasting time here seems quick, but as the meat has already been seared, it cooks through quickly in a hot oven.

The meat should be a little pink, but not raw: this is still pork, after all!
- I like to serve this with green beans, lightly steamed or boiled, and then tossed in a little Greek yogurt, salt and black pepper (100g = 35 cals).
- Why not try with baked hasselback potatoes: just carefully slice across the width of the potatoes at about 2mm intervals, rub with olive oil, season and bake for 1 hour at 180°C/gas mark 4 (1 medium-sized hasselback potato, approx. 150g = 135 calories).

Roast Asparagus with Grilled Halloumi, Orange & Almonds

This is such a simple but beautiful combination of flavours, and one of my favourite lunchtime dishes. It's probably a bit on the high side calorie-wise for a Light Day, but if it's a Regular Day, go right ahead – maybe even go for an extra slice of halloumi!

Quantity/serves: 2

Calories per serving: 349

Prep time: **15 mins**

Cooking time: **10 mins**

☒ Vegan   ☑ Lacto-Ovo Vegetarian

☒ Dairy-Free   ☑ Gluten-Free

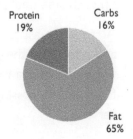

Protein 19% Carbs 16% Fat 65%

Ingredients

1 large orange, segmented (see Tips & Tweaks)
2 tsp white wine vinegar (or cider vinegar)
200g asparagus, woody ends trimmed
1 tsp extra-virgin olive oil
a pinch of salt
a pinch of freshly ground black pepper
150g halloumi cheese, cut into 1cm thick slices
15g (about 10) almonds, chopped

Method

Preheat the oven to 210°C/gas mark 6½.

Place the orange segments in a bowl with any retained juice and the vinegar. Place the asparagus on a roasting tray and rub with the olive oil. Season with the salt and pepper, then roast in the oven for 10 minutes.

Meanwhile, heat a large, non-stick frying pan or griddle pan over a medium heat. Add the halloumi to the pan and fry for 1–2 minutes on each side until golden.

Arrange the asparagus, halloumi and orange segments on a plate and pour over the orange juice and vinegar dressing. In a clean, dry frying pan over a medium heat, toast the chopped almonds for a few minutes, tossing occasionally. Sprinkle them over the top to serve.

Tips & Tweaks

- **How to segment an orange:** Using a sharp knife, carefully slice off the top and bottom of the orange. Using even, downward strokes, slice the skin away from the flesh and discard. Remove any remaining white pith. Cut between the membranes to segment the orange, retaining any juices for the dressing.
- This is best eaten straight away while the halloumi is warm, but you can make the rest of it in advance and then cook the cheese just before serving.

Sriracha Chicken Tray Bake with Charred Lemons

I didn't really know about sriracha until my son discovered it and started squirting it on everything! Well, if you can't beat them, join them – and I've found it makes a very simple and tasty marinade for chicken. So, if you have yet to try a bottle of this wonder-stuff, you are in for a treat.

Quantity/serves: 4

Calories per serving: 358

Prep time: 5 mins (plus marinating time)

Cooking time: 40 mins

☒ Vegan   ☒ Lacto-Ovo Vegetarian

☑ Dairy-Free   ☑ Gluten-Free

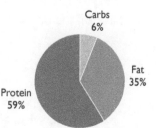

Carbs 6%

Fat 35%

Protein 59%

Ingredients

4 chicken legs (approx. 250g each), skin removed
1 lemon, thickly sliced
1 large red onion, thickly sliced

For the marinade
2 tbsp sriracha sauce
1 tbsp neutral oil
juice of ½ lemon
½ tsp ground cumin
½ tsp ground coriander
½ tsp mixed dried herbs

Method

Mix together the marinade ingredients in a large bowl. Add the chicken legs and toss well to coat. Cover with cling film and leave to marinate in the fridge (see Tips & Tweaks).

When you're ready to cook, preheat the oven to 220°C/gas mark 7. Place the lemon and red onion slices on the base of a roasting tin and arrange the chicken legs (smooth side up) on top. Spoon any excess marinade over the chicken. Roast for 30 minutes, turning the legs over every 10 minutes. Remove from the oven and give everything a good stir to release the onions and lemons from the base of the tin. Serve.

Tips & Tweaks

- Marinate the chicken for a few hours if you have time; otherwise, go straight in – it will still taste delicious.
- This is nice served with sourdough bread to mop up the pan juices (1 slice = 100 cals) and a green salad or some little baked potatoes (100g = 77 cals).

Crushed Potatoes with Peas, Smoked Salmon & Fried Egg

The recipe title tells you all you need to know, really. It's best made with pre-cooked potatoes, so if you fancy it for dinner, make sure to boil up the potatoes earlier in the day and leave them to cool. You can also use leftover potatoes if you happen to have some.

Quantity/serves: 2

Calories per serving: 365

Prep time: 5 mins

Cooking time: 15 mins

☒ Vegan   ☒ Lacto-Ovo Vegetarian

☑ Dairy-Free   ☑ Gluten-Free

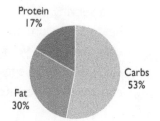

Protein 17%

Carbs 53%

Fat 30%

Ingredients

100g frozen peas
1 tbsp olive oil, plus extra if needed
1 small red onion, finely sliced
400g boiled potatoes with skins, crushed with a fork
a pinch of salt
a pinch of freshly ground black pepper
50g smoked salmon (approx. 2 slices), cut into ribbons
2 eggs

Method

Place the peas in a bowl and cover with boiling water from a kettle. Set aside to defrost.

Heat the oil in a large frying pan over a low heat. Add the onion and fry for 2–3 minutes until soft. Add the crushed potatoes and cook for 10 minutes more, or until they are starting to brown at the edges. Drain the peas and add them to the pan. Season well with salt and pepper and fry everything together for a further minute or two. Stir in the smoked salmon ribbons, then transfer the mixture to a serving plate. Return the frying pan to the hob, increase the heat to medium and add a drop more oil if needed. Crack in the eggs and fry to your liking (turning once if you prefer them over-easy). Place the eggs on top of the potato, pea and salmon mixture and serve immediately.

Tips & Tweaks

- If you have any chives or dill, snip some over the top for a fresh, herby garnish.

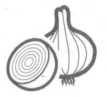

King Prawn & Pea Baked Biryani

This is a mildly spiced, baked rice dish that is really family-friendly: not too hot and super tasty. I use brown basmati rice for this – you could use white and reduce the cooking time by 20 minutes, but, of course, brown is healthier and has more fibre. You can make that call depending on your family's preferences!

Quantity/serves: 4

Calories per serving: 405

Prep time: **15 mins**

Cooking time: **60 mins**

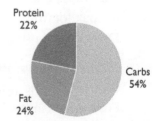

Protein 22%

Carbs 54%

Fat 24%

☒ Vegan   ☒ Lacto-Ovo Vegetarian

☒ Dairy-Free   ☑ Gluten-Free

Ingredients

250g brown basmati rice
200g frozen peas
300g raw king prawns
2 tbsp neutral oil
1 onion, sliced
3 garlic cloves, finely grated
3cm piece of fresh root ginger,
     peeled and finely grated
2 tsp mild curry powder
1 tsp garam masala
1 tsp ground cumin
1 tsp ground turmeric
1 small cinnamon stick
2 star anise
500ml hot vegetable stock, made from a cube

1 tsp butter
a good pinch of salt
a good pinch of freshly ground black pepper

Method

Preheat the oven to 180°C/gas mark 4.

Rinse the rice, then place in a bowl and cover with cold water. Put the frozen peas in a bowl of room-temperature water. If the prawns are frozen, do the same to defrost them prior to cooking. Leave all to soak for 10 minutes while you prep the rest of the ingredients. Drain before using.

In a large, ovenproof baking dish (preferably with a lid), mix together 1 tablespoon of the oil, the sliced onion and the garlic. Put the dish in the hot oven for 5 minutes, then take it out and add the remaining oil, along with the ginger, curry powder, garam masala, cumin and turmeric. Mix well and return to the oven for a further 5 minutes. Remove from the oven again and this time add the drained peas and prawns, along with the cinnamon stick and star anise. Give everything a good stir, then spoon the drained rice evenly over the top. In a jug, mix together the stock, butter, salt and pepper, stirring to dissolve the butter. Pour the stock carefully over the rice. Place the lid on the baking dish (if you don't have a lid, you could use foil, but you might have to weigh it down if you have a fan-assisted oven). Bake for 45 minutes.

Take the dish out of the oven and give everything a gentle stir. Taste the rice and, if it still has too much bite, spread it back out, sprinkle over a few tablespoons of water (if needed) and cook for a further 5 minutes or so. Once the rice is fully cooked, give it a stir to incorporate any juices still at the bottom of the dish and put the lid or foil back on for a few minutes so the final juices can be absorbed. Remove the cinnamon stick and star anise before serving.

Tips & Tweaks

- You can make this recipe up to the point where the stock is added, then cover it with a lid or foil and pop it in the fridge until you're ready to bake.
- If easier, you can do the first stage on the hob, using an ovenproof casserole which can go in the oven once you've added the rice and stock.
- Other suggestions to add even more flavour: swirl in some Greek yogurt (1 tbsp = 15 cals); chop over a few mint leaves; or squeeze over some fresh lemon juice.

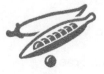

Easy Spinach & Ricotta Wholewheat Cannelloni

If you have family members who don't mind giving a hand in the kitchen (lucky you!), then this one is great to set them to work on. You need to have some Rich Tomato Sauce (p. 128) made up in advance, but other than that, it's child's play.

Quantity/serves: 4

Calories per serving: 425

Prep time: **15 mins**

Cooking time: **35 mins**

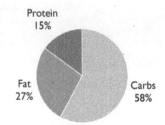

☒ Vegan   ☑ Lacto-Ovo Vegetarian

☒ Dairy-Free   ☒ Gluten-Free

Ingredients

1 tsp olive oil
16 sheets wholewheat lasagne
200g spinach leaves
250g ricotta cheese
1 tsp lemon juice
a pinch of salt
a pinch of freshly ground black pepper
350g Rich Tomato Sauce
50g mature Cheddar cheese, grated

Method

Preheat the oven to 180°C/gas mark 4.

Put a large saucepan of salted water over a medium heat and add the olive oil. Bring to the boil. When bubbling, add the lasagne sheets, adding them one by one to prevent sticking. Reduce the heat to low and cook for about 5 minutes, until pliable but not fully cooked. Drain the pasta and place it in a bowl of cold water to cool, then drain again and separate out the sheets so they are ready to use.

Meanwhile, place the spinach, ricotta and lemon juice in a food processor and blitz. Season well with salt and pepper.

Spread half of the tomato sauce over the base of a large baking dish. Now, taking each lasagne sheet in turn, spoon some of the spinach and ricotta mixture along the length of one side and roll up to make a cigar shape. Line them up in the baking dish, cover with the rest of the tomato sauce and top with the grated Cheddar. Bake for 25–30 minutes, or until the cheese is bubbling and golden.

Tips & Tweaks

- Serve with a peppery, rocket salad (100g = 25 cals).
- Adjust your serving size according to whether it's a Light Day or a Regular Day: each cannelloni is approx. 106 cals, so have 2–3 on a Light Day and 4 on a Regular Day.

Simple Chicken Chasseur

I've been making this pared-down chicken chasseur for years, and can't for the life of me remember where the original recipe came from, but it's a corker. It's so rich and tasty. It's absolutely delicious on a Regular Day served with a large dish of blanched green vegetables and some creamy mash.

Quantity/serves: 4

Calories per serving: 435

Prep time: 10 mins

Cooking time: 60–80 mins

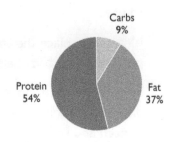

Carbs 9%
Protein 54%
Fat 37%

☒ Vegan   ☒ Lacto-Ovo Vegetarian

☒ Dairy-Free   ☑ Gluten-Free

Ingredients

1 tsp olive oil
20g butter
4 chicken legs (approx. 250g each), skin removed
a pinch of salt
a pinch of freshly ground black pepper
1 onion, chopped
2 garlic cloves, crushed
200g small button mushrooms, left whole or halved
    depending on size
225ml red wine
2 tbsp tomato purée
2 thyme sprigs
500ml chicken stock, made from a cube

Method

Heat the oil and half of the butter in a deep, lidded frying pan or casserole over a medium heat. Season the chicken legs with salt and pepper and add them to the pan. Fry for about 5 minutes on each side until golden brown. Remove from the pan and set aside.

With the pan still on the heat, add the remaining butter and melt. Add the onion and fry for about 5 minutes until soft. Add the garlic and cook for about 1 minute, then add the mushrooms and cook for 2 minutes more. Now stir in the wine, followed by the tomato purée. Let it bubble and reduce for about 5 minutes, then stir in the thyme sprigs and pour over the stock. Return the chicken legs to the pan, cover with a lid and simmer over a low heat for 1 hour until the chicken is very tender, stirring and turning the legs over occasionally.

Remove the chicken from the pan, place on a plate and cover with foil to keep warm. Increase the heat to high and reduce the sauce on a rapid boil for about 10 minutes. Return the chicken legs to the sauce and serve.

Tips & Tweaks

- You can make this dish in advance and reheat it when it's time to eat: the flavours are even better that way.
- I usually serve this with green beans (100g = 31 cals). Some other good options are white cabbage (100g = 25 cals), some crusty bread (1 slice = 100 cals) or crushed new potatoes (100g = 77 cals).
- This is a perfect dish to serve when you have friends over.

Lamb Curry Fake-away

Fancy a takeaway curry? Well, save yourself some money (and calories!) and cook this up instead. Make it in the morning so it has time to simmer away for a few hours, then in the evening, just heat it up and devour. It's like getting a delivery from your local Indian restaurant, but healthier!

Quantity/serves: 4

Calories per serving: 452

Prep time: 15 mins

Cooking time: 2–3 hours

☒ Vegan   ☒ Lacto-Ovo Vegetarian

☑ Dairy-Free   ☑ Gluten-Free

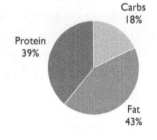

Protein 39%
Carbs 18%
Fat 43%

Ingredients

1 tbsp neutral oil
750g lamb, cubed, any excess fat trimmed
1 onion, finely chopped
2 garlic cloves, finely grated
3cm piece of fresh root ginger, finely grated
1 tsp ground cumin
1 tbsp garam masala
1 tsp chilli powder (or to taste)
6 cardamom pods, lightly crushed
1 small cinnamon stick
2 tbsp tomato purée
500ml vegetable stock, made from a cube
2 × 400g cans plum tomatoes
a good pinch of salt

Method

Heat the oil in a large saucepan over a medium heat. Add the lamb and fry for 4–5 minutes until it is brown all over, then pour off any excess fat. Add the onion and fry for a couple of minutes, then stir in the garlic and ginger. Add all the spices, including the cinnamon stick, and fry for another minute or so. Stir in the tomato purée, stock, tomatoes and salt, then cover the pan with a lid and simmer for 2–3 hours until the meat is tender. Check and stir occasionally to break up the tomatoes, adding more water if it seems to be getting too dry: you are looking for a thick-ish curry sauce consistency. This can be served straight away, or will keep in the fridge for up to 3 days.

Tips & Tweaks

- This curry needs a good couple of hours of simmering for the lamb to really become tender. You could also make it the day before.
- You can cook this in the oven rather than simmer it on the hob. Prepare it in an ovenproof casserole and transfer it to the oven to cook. It will take 2–3 hours at 160°C/gas mark 3 – remember to check it every so often to give it a stir and add a little water if necessary.
- Serve with some Greek yogurt (1 tbsp = 15 cals), brown basmati rice (100g cooked weight = 110 cals) or homemade flatbreads (p. 156; 1 flatbread = 100 cals).

Smoked Mackerel Bowl with Avocado & Curried Lentils

I'd be hard pushed to get more of my favourite ingredients and flavours into one bowl. To be honest, once I had the idea for this in my head, I was like a thing possessed; I made a special trip to the shops to get the smoked mackerel and find the perfect avocado, just so I could have it for lunch. I hope you feel similarly inspired!

Quantity/serves: 2

Calories per serving: 494

Prep time: **15 mins**

Cooking time: **20 mins**

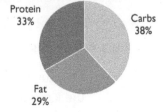

Protein 33%
Carbs 38%
Fat 29%

☒ Vegan ☒ Lacto-Ovo Vegetarian

☒ Dairy-Free ☑ Gluten-Free

Ingredients

125g dried green, brown, puy or beluga lentils
1 egg
2 tbsp Greek yogurt
1 tsp mild curry powder
a pinch of salt
a pinch of freshly ground black pepper
2 smoked mackerel fillets (approx. 75g each),
    skin removed, flesh flaked
4 spring onions, sliced
a handful of cherry tomatoes, halved
½ avocado, sliced
½ lemon, cut into two wedges
a few sprigs of coriander

Method

Place the lentils in a saucepan of unsalted water over a medium heat and bring to the boil. Reduce the heat to low and simmer for 20 minutes until tender.

Meanwhile, bring another saucepan of water to the boil over a high heat. Carefully lower in the egg, then reduce the heat to low and simmer for 7 minutes (for medium-boiled – add an extra couple of minutes if you prefer the yolk completely solid).

In a small bowl, mix together the yogurt and curry powder and season well with salt and pepper. When the lentils are cooked, rinse with cold water to cool them down and drain well. Dress the lentils with the yogurt mixture and divide between two bowls. Cool, peel and halve the boiled egg. Now arrange the mackerel, spring onions, cherry tomatoes and avocado on top of the lentils, and finish each bowl with half an egg, a lemon wedge and a sprig of coriander.

Tips & Tweaks

- You can freeze smoked mackerel, so I always have a couple of packs in the freezer ready for a quick meal.
- To make this even easier, just use a 250g pouch of pre-cooked lentils.
- This is a lovely one to make if you have people coming over for lunch: it looks so pretty and it's delicious.

Salmon Tray Bake with Pak Choi & Noodles

Everyone loves a tray bake – one tin, virtually no effort and maximum flavour. I wanted to make something really family-friendly and, assuming your family like salmon, this is a winner. You can also serve this on a Light Day – just avoid the noodles. On a Regular Day, get stuck in with the rest of the family.

Quantity/serves: 4

Calories per serving (with noodles): 520

Protein 27%
Carbs 35%
Fat 38%

Calories per serving (without noodles): 298

Carbs 13%
Protein 38%
Fat 49%

Prep time: **10 mins**

Cooking time: **30 mins**

☒ Vegan   ☒ Lacto-Ovo Vegetarian

☑ Dairy-Free   ☑ Gluten-Free (use tamari)

Ingredients

> 4 salmon fillets (approx. 120g each)
> 2 tbsp salt dissolved in approx. 500ml cold water
> 200g dried fine egg noodles
> 1 tbsp sesame oil
> 300g pak choi, cut into long strips
> 3 tbsp soy sauce (use tamari for GF)

1 tbsp runny honey
juice of 2 limes
4cm piece of fresh root ginger, peeled and cut into
    thick sticks
1 large red chilli, deseeded and sliced

Method

Preheat the oven to 180°C/gas mark 4.

Place the salmon fillets in a large bowl and pour over the salted water. Leave to brine for 10 minutes – this will prevent the fillets from oozing white stuff when they cook.

Meanwhile, cook the noodles according to the packet instructions, then drain and toss with the sesame oil. Place the noodles in a baking dish (ideally one with a lid) and cover with the pak choi. Position the brined salmon fillets on top.

In a small bowl, mix together the soy sauce, honey, lime juice and 3 tablespoons water. Pour half of this mixture over the salmon fillets. Top the fillets with the chopped ginger and chilli (if you have anyone in your family who doesn't like heat, just leave the chilli off their piece of fish). Place the lid on the baking dish or cover with foil, making sure it's a snug fit so the salmon steams as well as bakes. Bake for 20 minutes, then pour the remaining soy mixture over the fish before serving.

Tips & Tweaks

*   You can get everything ready in the tray earlier in the day, then cover with the lid or with foil and keep in the fridge until it's time to cook.

Tandoori Whole Roast Chicken with Spicy Potatoes

Here's a lovely new take on roast chicken for the weekend, although I have made this on a weekday before. If it's a Light Day, I skip the potatoes and remove the skin, and have with lots of green veg.

Quantity/serves: 4

Calories per serving (with skin & potatoes): 683

Calories per serving (without skin & potatoes): 364

Protein 32%
Carbs 23%
Fat 45%

Carbs 2%
Fat 35%
Protein 63%

Prep time: **10 mins** (plus optional marinating time)

Cooking time: **60 mins**

☒ Vegan   ☒ Lacto-Ovo Vegetarian

☑ Dairy-Free   ☑ Gluten-Free

Ingredients

1 whole chicken (approx. 1.2kg)
4 potatoes, cut into wedges lengthways
1 tsp olive oil
a pinch of salt
a pinch of freshly ground black pepper
1 lemon, cut into 4 wedges

For the spice paste
2 tbsp neutral oil
1 tsp ground ginger
1 tsp ground cumin
1 tsp ground coriander
1 tsp paprika
1 tsp turmeric
½ tsp salt
½ tsp cayenne pepper (optional – it's spicy!)

Method

Preheat the oven to 200°C/gas mark 6.

Make the spice paste by combining all the ingredients in a bowl. Place the chicken in a large roasting tin, prick the skin all over with the tip of a sharp knife, then slather the spice paste all over the chicken (see Tips & Tweaks). Rub the potato wedges with a little olive oil, salt and pepper and arrange around the chicken. Tuck the lemon wedges in alongside the potatoes. Roast for 50 minutes, then take the tray out of the oven and remove the potatoes to a serving dish, covering it with foil to keep them warm. Increase the oven temperature to 220°C/gas mark 7 and put the chicken back in for a final 10 minutes to let the skin crisp up.

Tips & Tweaks

- If you have time, leave the chicken with the spice paste on to marinate for a few hours before roasting.
- Note that the chicken should be at room temperature for roasting: if it's cold from the fridge, it will take longer.
- Pour any juices from the roasting tin into a jug and use as gravy.
- Have this with a big green salad, or perhaps the Beetroot, Carrot & Apple Slaw (p. 134). You could also serve with a simple yogurt and cucumber raita (1 heaped tbsp = 20 cals).

SWEET STUFF & SNACKS

Healthy Peanut Choc Chip Energy Bites

I have borrowed the flavours of a well-known chocolate bar here (peanuts, salt, chocolate) to create what I think might be the most delicious healthy snack ever. And the best thing? You don't even need to cook them: just keep in the freezer, ready for when the munchies call.

Quantity/serves: 24 bites

Calories per bite: 100

Prep time: 15 mins

Cooking time: 0 mins

☑ Vegan   ☑ Lacto-Ovo Vegetarian

☑ Dairy-Free   ☑ Gluten-Free (use GF oats)

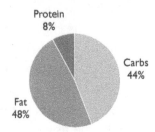

Ingredients

      75g roasted, salted peanuts
      50g raw cashew nuts, unsalted
      100g rolled oats
      5 Medjool dates, pitted
      3 soft dried figs
      10g sunflower seeds
      10g chia seeds
      2 tbsp coconut oil
      2 tbsp date syrup (or other sweetener like maple
        syrup)
      75g good-quality dark chocolate chips

Method

Line a 15 × 20cm tin with a strip of baking parchment, leaving the ends poking out so it's easy to lift out of the tin later.

Roughly chop half the peanuts and cashews and set aside. Put the rest of the nuts and the oats into a blender or food processor and blitz to a breadcrumb texture. Add the dates and figs and blend until fairly uniform in appearance (no big lumps of fruit). Place the mixture in a large bowl. Add the seeds and the reserved chopped nuts and mix well to combine.

In a small saucepan over a low heat, gently heat the oil and date syrup for a minute or so until runny, then pour into the nut mixture. Combine well and leave to cool (you can pop it in the fridge for a few minutes if you like). Now add the chocolate chips and stir through to distribute evenly. Press the mixture into the prepared tin and place in the freezer for an hour or so to firm up. Remove from the tin and cut into 24 bite-sized squares.

Tips & Tweaks

- You can be flexible with the ingredients: if you don't have cashews, use almonds or another nut. The seeds can be changed up, too.
- Store in the freezer in an airtight container with baking parchment between the layers to stop the bites sticking together. You can eat these straight from frozen.

Anoeska's Chococo Clusters

Thanks to my friend Anoeska for donating this recipe. She is not only one of the healthiest people I know, but also speaks a gazillion languages fluently. If these are good enough for Anoeska, they are good enough for me!

Quantity/serves: makes 20 × 20g clusters

Calories per cluster: 129

Prep time: **5 mins**

Cooking time: **10 mins**

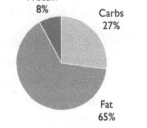

☑ Vegan   ☑ Lacto-Ovo Vegetarian

☑ Dairy-Free (ensure dark chocolate is milk-free)

☑ Gluten-Free

Ingredients

　　　200g flaked almonds
　　　1 tsp coconut oil
　　　200g dark chocolate (70%+ cocoa solids), broken up
　　　50g dried cranberries
　　　1 tbsp unsweetened desiccated coconut (optional)
　　　a pinch of sea salt flakes

Method

Line a baking sheet with baking parchment.

Place a large frying pan over a medium heat. Add the flaked almonds and toast them carefully until they are just starting to brown: do not burn, or they will go very bitter. Take off the heat and set aside.

Place a saucepan of water over a medium heat. Set a large, heatproof bowl over the hot water (this is known as a bain-marie). Place the coconut oil and broken-up chocolate in the bowl, and keep stirring until melted. Add the toasted almonds, along with the dried cranberries and desiccated coconut, and mix everything until well combined. Then place spoonfuls of the mixture on to the prepared baking sheet. For portion control, this recipe makes 20 clusters of approximately 20g each. Lightly sprinkle sea salt flakes over the top, then put in the fridge to set. Once cooled, peel the clusters off the baking parchment and keep them in an airtight container in the fridge. They will keep in the fridge for at least 2–3 weeks (but they're so tasty, they probably won't hang around that long!).

Tips & Tweaks

- You can substitute raisins if you don't have any dried cranberries.
- These make a sophisticated after-dinner treat if you have guests over.
- Why not use up some of those spare Regular Day calories and have one of these if you need a sweet hit?

Black Bean Brownies

I cannot take the credit for this recipe. I discovered it on @flavourforager's Instagram page, but it has since become a firm favourite and so I had to include it here. The first time I made these, I didn't tell the kids what was in them due to their bean aversion. They gobbled them up – indeed, there were even 'mmmmm' sounds! So, if you are looking for a healthy bake or a sweet treat on a Regular Day, then look no further.

Quantity/serves: 9 brownies

Calories per brownie: 147

Prep time: 10 mins

Cooking time: 20 mins

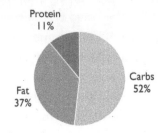

☒ Vegan ☑ Lacto-Ovo Vegetarian

☑ Dairy-Free ☑ Gluten-Free

Ingredients

400g can black beans, drained and rinsed
3 eggs
3 tbsp neutral oil
25g unsweetened cocoa powder
115g golden caster sugar
½ tsp baking powder
a good pinch of salt

Method

Preheat the oven to 180°C/gas mark 4 and line a small 15cm square baking tray with baking parchment (use one piece and fold it into the corners: that way you can easily lift the brownies out once they're cool).

Place the beans, eggs and oil in a food processor and blitz until completely blended. In a separate bowl, combine the dry ingredients, then add them to the food processor. Pulse everything together until combined, then pour the batter into the prepared tin. Bake for 20 minutes. Allow the brownies to cool in the tin before cutting into 9 squares.

Tips & Tweaks

- These make a sensational Regular Day dessert paired with Banana Nicecream (p. 248).

Poached Passion Fruit Pears

This is a beautifully simple and healthy dessert that works equally well served with creamy Greek yogurt for breakfast on a Light Day, or with a scoop of vanilla ice cream for dessert on a Regular Day!

Quantity/serves: 4

Calories per serving: 204

Prep time: 10 mins

Cooking time: 25–35 mins

☑ Vegan   ☑ Lacto-Ovo Vegetarian

☑ Dairy-Free   ☑ Gluten-Free

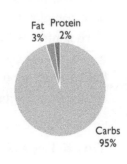

Fat 3%   Protein 2%   Carbs 95%

Ingredients

750ml clear apple juice
pulp of 3 passion fruit
1 star anise (optional)
1 bay leaf (optional)
4 slightly under-ripe pears
juice of ½ lemon

Method

Place the apple juice, passion fruit pulp, star anise and bay leaf in a saucepan over a medium heat and bring to the boil. Meanwhile, peel the pears and rub them with a little lemon juice to stop them browning. Place the pears in the pan, along with the remaining lemon juice, and reduce the heat to a simmer. Cook for 25–35 minutes, turning occasionally, until the pears are tender when tested with a sharp knife. Remove the pears from the poaching liquid and set aside. Increase the heat to high and boil the liquid vigorously for around 3 minutes to reduce further. Pour the sauce into a jug to serve alongside the pears. These can be eaten hot or cold.

Tips & Tweaks

- These can be made in advance and stored in the fridge for several days.
- I love eating these cold from the fridge with yogurt in the morning. On a Regular Day, I'll add a sprinkling of My Go-to Granola (p. 89) too.

Baked Stone Fruits with Spiced Yogurt

This is a lovely seasonal recipe. When those gorgeous stone fruits – peaches, nectarines, plums and apricots – come in to season in the summer months, buy a bunch of punnets and make this for delicious, healthy desserts or to use as a chunky compote served with yogurt and granola.

Quantity/serves: 4

Calories per serving: 205

Prep time: 10 mins

Cooking time: 20 mins

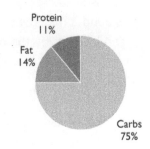

☒ Vegan   ☑ Lacto-Ovo Vegetarian

☒ Dairy-Free   ☑ Gluten-Free

Ingredients

   1kg stone fruits (peaches, nectarines, plums and
      apricots), halved and stoned
4 tbsp (60ml) honey
juice of 1 lemon
100ml Greek yogurt
1 tsp icing sugar (optional)
½ tsp mixed spice
20g flaked almonds

Method

Preheat the oven to 200°C/gas mark 6.

Place the fruit halves, cut-side up, in a baking dish. In a small bowl, whisk together the honey, lemon juice and 2 tablespoons water with a fork. Pour this mixture over the fruit, then place the baking dish in the hot oven. Check after 15 minutes: the fruit should be tender, but not completely disintegrating. If the fruit is sufficiently baked, take the dish out of the oven; if not, leave for another 5 minutes or so. The ripeness of the fruit will affect how long it takes.

While the fruit is cooking, mix together the yogurt, icing sugar (if using) and mixed spice in a bowl and set aside. Then place a small frying pan over a medium heat and toast the flaked almonds for about 1 minute until just turning golden, being careful not to burn them.

Serve the fruit straight from the baking dish and top with the toasted almonds and spiced yogurt.

Tips & Tweaks

- If you have some of My Go-to Granola made up (p. 89; 100g granola = 412 cals), you can sprinkle some over the top before baking the fruit for a healthy take on a fruit crumble.

Roasted Figs with Dark Chocolate Drizzle

My take on sweet things these days is to use the naturally occurring sugar in fruit wherever possible. These rather delicious roasted figs are a case in point. I do add a little brown sugar, and there's some dark chocolate, too, but the syrupy sauce is mainly sweetened with orange juice. With a spoonful of mascarpone, this makes a lovely dessert for when you have people over.

Quantity/serves: 4

Calories per serving: 212

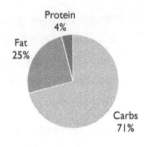

Prep time: **5 mins**

Cooking time: **25 mins**

☑ Vegan (ensure dark chocolate is milk-free and wine is certified vegan)

☑ Lacto-Ovo Vegetarian

☑ Dairy-Free (ensure dark chocolate is milk-free)

☑ Gluten-Free

Ingredients

250ml red wine
juice of 1 large orange
2 tbsp dark brown sugar
½ cinnamon stick
8 fresh figs, halved
40g dark chocolate
    (70%+ cocoa solids),
    broken up

Method

Preheat the oven to 170°C/gas mark 3½.

Place the red wine, orange juice, sugar and cinnamon stick in a small saucepan over a high heat and boil fairly vigorously until the mixture has reduced down to about half its original volume (this will take about 10 minutes).

Place the halved figs in a small baking tin or dish and pour over the red wine syrup. Place in the oven and bake for 15 minutes.

Meanwhile, place a saucepan of water over a medium heat and bring to a gentle simmer. Set a heatproof bowl over the hot water. Add the chocolate to the bowl and let it slowly melt.

Remove the figs from the oven and place in a pretty serving bowl. Pour over the syrup from the baking dish and, using a metal spoon, drizzle some melted chocolate over each fig.

Tips & Tweaks

- These are best eaten straight away, while still warm.
- Some soft mascarpone cheese is a lovely addition (1 tbsp = 122 cals), or use Greek yogurt for a lower-cal option (1 tbsp = 15 cals).

Mango Chia Cheesecake

This is a brilliant dessert to whip out when people come over for dinner, because it's one of those 'I can't believe this is low-cal' recipes. It's also spectacularly easy to make and sits quite happily in the fridge for a day or two, which ticks all my boxes when it comes to a dinner party pud.

Quantity/serves: 4

Calories per serving: 242

Prep time: 15 mins
(plus at least 3 hours chilling)

Cooking time: 0 mins

Protein 17%

Carbs 50%

Fat 33%

☒ Vegan   ☑ Lacto-Ovo Vegetarian

☒ Dairy-Free   ☑ Gluten-Free (use GF oatcakes)

Ingredients

For the base
4 (approx. 50g total) shop-bought rough oatcakes
20g butter or coconut oil
2 tsp maple syrup
½ tsp ground ginger
½ tsp ground cinnamon

For the filling
250ml Greek yogurt
50g chia seeds
2 tsp maple syrup
½ tsp vanilla extract

For the topping
250g fresh or frozen mango (or other fruit of your
    choice: berries work well, too)
zest of 1 lime

Method

Place the oatcakes in a resealable bag or similar and, pressing down firmly with a rolling pin, crush until they form a fine crumb.

In a small saucepan over a low heat, gently melt the butter (or coconut oil). Remove from the heat and add the maple syrup to the pan, followed by the oatcake crumbs, and the ginger and cinnamon. Mix well to combine. Press the mixture into the bases of 4 ramekins or small glasses and place in the fridge for at least half an hour to cool.

Meanwhile, combine the yogurt, chia seeds, maple syrup and vanilla extract in a bowl. When the bases have cooled, spoon the yogurt filling over the top. Return the ramekins or glasses to the fridge to chill for at least 3 hours, or overnight if possible, so that the chia seeds have time to expand and set.

To make the fruit topping, blitz up the mango in a food processor or blender (if you're using frozen mango, let it defrost a little bit first to soften). Spoon the fruity purée over the chia cheesecake filling and grate fresh lime zest over the top to finish. Serve immediately.

Tips & Tweaks

- Make everything in advance and keep it in the fridge until you're ready, except the fruity topping, which you can add just before serving.
- Remove from the fridge 10 minutes before adding the fruit purée and serving, so it can soften a little.
- To make one large cheesecake to serve 8 people, just double the quantities and use a 20cm springform tin.

Apple & Raspberry Cake

On a Regular Day, when you have more calories to play with, you may well fancy a slice of cake, but we all know that it doesn't deliver so much on the nutritional front. So, I've come up with this: a cake that tastes great, but has plenty of fruit and less sugar and butter, so it won't undo all that good work you've done on your Light Days.

Quantity/serves: 8

Calories per serving: 269

Prep time: **15 mins**

Cooking time: **40 mins**

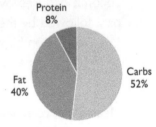

Protein 8%
Carbs 52%
Fat 40%

☒ Vegan   ☑ Lacto-Ovo Vegetarian

☒ Dairy-Free   ☒ Gluten-Free

Ingredients

150g fresh raspberries
1 tsp icing sugar
200g wholemeal self-raising flour
   (or add 2½ tsp baking powder to wholemeal plain flour)
2 tsp ground cinnamon
100g cold unsalted butter, diced
100g light brown sugar
2 eggs
1 tsp vanilla extract
125ml semi-skimmed milk
150g eating apples (approx. 2 apples),
   peeled, cored and grated

Method

Preheat the oven to 160°C/gas mark 3 and grease and flour a 20cm cake tin.

Place the raspberries in a large mixing bowl with the icing sugar and mix well, crushing the fruit a little with a fork.

Place the flour and cinnamon in a food processor and pulse to combine. Now add the butter and pulse again a few times until the mixture resembles breadcrumbs. Add the sugar and pulse until mixed in. Whisk the eggs, vanilla and milk together in a jug. With the food processor on a low setting, slowly pour in the egg mixture until just combined.

Pour this mixture into the bowl with the raspberries, then add the grated apples and stir everything together well. Pour the batter into the prepared tin and bake for 40 minutes. A metal skewer poked into the middle should come out clean. Allow to cool for at least 10 minutes before taking the cake out of the tin.

Tips & Tweaks

- You can substitute fresh blueberries for raspberries in this recipe if you prefer.
- Serve with some Greek yogurt (1 tbsp = 15 cals).

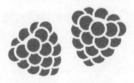

Banana Nicecream

The idea of making a quick ice cream out of frozen bananas isn't anything new, but it's well worth rediscovering because it's a brilliantly quick and healthy treat. You can experiment with your own flavour combos: I've given two of my favourites.

Quantity/serves: 2

Calories per serving: 151

Prep time: 5 mins

Cooking time: 0 mins

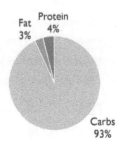

Fat 3%
Protein 4%
Carbs 93%

☑ Vegan (ensure chocolate chips are vegan if using)

☑ Lacto-Ovo Vegetarian   ☑ Dairy-Free   ☑ Gluten-Free

Ingredients

Plain
2 large ripe bananas, peeled, chopped and frozen (approx. 300g)

Variations

- Chocolate Chip & Peanut Butter (306 cals per serving): 25g dark chocolate chips, 2 tbsp crunchy peanut butter
- Rum & Raisin (239 cals per serving): 50ml dark rum, 30g raisins

Method

For plain banana nicecream, place the frozen banana chunks in a food processor or blender and blitz until smooth. You'll need to do this on high, and scrape down the sides a few times.

For the chocolate chip and peanut butter variation, add the peanut butter to the food processor at the same time as the banana and blitz, then add the chocolate chips and just pulse once or twice to combine, or stir in by hand.

For the rum and raisin variation, heat the rum and the raisins in a small saucepan over a low heat until warm, then take off the heat and let soak for 15 minutes. Pour any residual rum into the food processor with the bananas and blitz, then add the raisins and just pulse once or twice to combine, or stir in by hand.

Serve immediately, or transfer to a container and freeze for half an hour, then scoop out with an ice cream scoop.

Tips & Tweaks

- The bananas need to be frozen overnight before using. It's best to use very ripe bananas, then peel and slice before freezing.
- Another lovely combination is banana and frozen berries.

Ten Light Day Meal Combos

All the meal combos in this section have been put together to come in under the Light Day allowance of 800 calories and be nutritionally balanced. Any spare calories are indicated and can be used as you wish – perhaps on some extra vegetables with a meal, or a splash of milk here and there in tea and coffee. On Light Days you don't have many calories to play with, so it's best to avoid alcohol and snacks.

The combos give suggestions for three meals a day, but for many of us it's not practical to cook this often. You can easily make something like a soup, curry or stew stretch over two days or longer by making double the quantity.

You can, if you prefer, put together your own Light Day combos using the recipes in this book, or if you have other low-calorie favourites, by all means include some of those. You just have to make sure your calorie total for the day comes in under 800.

In the Resources section at the end of the book I have given some of my favourite cookbooks and websites for low-calorie recipes.

	LIGHT DAY COMBO 1		
		Cals/serving	*Page*
Breakfast	Oaty Miracle Muffins	167	93
Lunch	Indian Black Bean & Spinach Soup	233	168
Dinner	Teriyaki Mackerel with Sesame Spinach	267	182

Total calories: **667**

Spare calories: **133**

LIGHT DAY COMBO 2

		Cals/serving	Page
Breakfast	Apple & Carrot Basic Bircher	182	95
Lunch	Broccerino Soup	173	144
Dinner	Best Black Bean Chilli	230	166

Total calories: **585**

Spare calories: 215

LIGHT DAY COMBO 3

		Cals/serving	Page
Breakfast	The Healthiest Pancakes in the World	160	87
	with Quick Berry Sauce	39	86
Lunch	Carrot, Lemon & Ginger Soup	186	146
Dinner	Flaky Curried Fish with one Flatbread	242	172

Total calories: **627**

Spare calories: 173

LIGHT DAY COMBO 4

		Cals/serving	Page
Breakfast	Big Mushrooms	210	103
Lunch	Green Lentil, Tomato & Watercress Soup	164	138
Dinner	Fast Fish Pie	278	186

Total calories: **652**

Spare calories: 148

LIGHT DAY COMBO 5

		Cals/serving	Page
Breakfast	Indian Spiced Omelette Wrap	167	91
Lunch	Potato, Leek & Fennel Soup with Stilton	191	150
Dinner	Simple Veggie Tagine	224	164

Total calories: **582**

Spare calories: 218

LIGHT DAY COMBO 6

		Cals/serving	Page
Breakfast	Baked Bacon & Eggs with Asparagus Dippers	194	99
Lunch	Rainbow Ribbon Salad with a Tahini Dressing	235	170
Dinner	Tagliata & Watercress with a Mustard Orange Dressing	289	190

Total calories: **718**

Spare calories: 82

LIGHT DAY COMBO 7

		Cals/serving	Page
Breakfast	Brilliant Breakfast Muffins	193	97
Lunch	Beans Provençale	210	162
Dinner	Roast Cod with Basil Sauce & Cherry Tomatoes	186	148

Total calories: **589**

Spare calories: 211

The Recipes

LIGHT DAY COMBO 8

		Cals/serving	Page
Breakfast	Chorizo Omelette	208	101
Lunch	Tasty Tuna Toast Topper	208	160
Dinner	'They'll Never Know' Veggie Ragu, served with 100g (cooked weight) of wholegrain spaghetti	223	132

Total calories: **639**

Spare calories: 161

LIGHT DAY COMBO 9

		Cals/serving	Page
Breakfast	Cream Cheese, Smoked Salmon, Lemon & Red Onion (on toast)	184	119
Lunch	Spinach & Parmesan Crustless Quiche	196	154
Dinner	Broccoli, Bacon & Cheddar Burgers	160	136

Total calories: **540**

Spare calories: 260

LIGHT DAY COMBO 10

		Cals/serving	Page
Breakfast	Any 'Breakfast & brunch' recipe under 200 cals	200	80
Lunch	Any Quick Lunch Assembly under 300 cals	300	196–9
Dinner	Any meal recipe under 300 cals per serving	300	80–3

Total calories: **800**

Ten Regular Day Meal Combos

On Regular Days we have more calories to play with, so the focus is on good nutrition rather than weight loss. The meal combos I've put together here all come in well under the Regular Day calorie allowances of 1,600 for a woman and 2,000 for a man, so you have some flexibility.

You could increase your portion size a bit if you are feeling particularly hungry, add some tasty side dishes (suggested sides are given for most of the recipes) or use up the spare calories with healthy snacks, a sweet treat (I have given suggestions for you to try) or perhaps have that flat white or a glass of wine.

Here are my suggested Regular Day Meal Combos. Please feel free to make up your own based on the recipes you're particularly drawn to.

REGULAR DAY COMBO 1			
		Cals/serving	Page
Breakfast	Power-through Porridges	256	107
Lunch	Baked Sweet Potatoes with Tzatziki	299	192
Dinner	Simple Chicken Chasseur	435	222
	Total calories: **990**		
	Spare calories: **610** woman / **1,010** man		
Why not try	Mango Chia Cheesecake	242	244

The Recipes

REGULAR DAY COMBO 2

		Cals/serving	Page
Breakfast	Nut Butter, Banana & Cinnamon (on toast)	257	118
Lunch	Vietnamese-Style Chicken Salad	246	174
Dinner	Smoked Mackerel Bowl with Avocado & Curried Lentils	494	226

Total calories: **997**

Spare calories: 603 woman / **1,003** man

Why not try	Anoeska's Chococo Clusters	129	234

REGULAR DAY COMBO 3

		Cals/serving	Page
Breakfast	Simple Smoothie Bowl	284	109
Lunch	Warm Spinach Salad with Feta & Strawberries	277	184
Dinner	Sriracha Chicken Tray Bake with Charred Lemons	358	213

Total calories: **919**

Spare calories: 681 woman / **1,081** man

Why not try	Black Bean Brownies	147	236

REGULAR DAY COMBO 4

		Cals/serving	Page
Breakfast	Spinachy Baked Eggs	242	105
Lunch	Crushed Potatoes with Peas, Smoked Salmon & Fried Egg	365	215
Dinner	Easy Spinach & Ricotta Wholewheat Cannelloni	425	220

Total calories: **1032**

Spare calories: 568 woman / **968** man

Why not try	Healthy Peanut Choc Chip Energy Bites	100	232

REGULAR DAY COMBO 5

		Cals/serving	Page
Breakfast	Mexican Breakfast Bowl	312	111
Lunch	Spinach, Mushroom, Onion & Feta Flatbreads	200	156
Dinner	King Prawn & Pea Baked Biryani	405	217

Total calories: **917**

Spare calories: 683 woman / 1,083 man

Why not try	Rum & Raisin Banana Nicecream	239	248

REGULAR DAY COMBO 6

		Cals/serving	Page
Breakfast	Oatcakes with Tomato, Avocado & Feta	268	116
Lunch	Puy Lentil & Tomato Salad with Goat's Cheese & Green Chilli	315	204
Dinner	Salmon Tray Bake with Pak Choi & Noodles	520	228

Total calories: **1103**

Spare calories: 497 woman / 897 man

Why not try	Chocolate Chip & Peanut Butter Banana Nicecream	306	248

REGULAR DAY COMBO 7

		Cals/serving	Page
Breakfast	Brekkie in a Hurry	317	113
Lunch	Pot Noodles	260	180
Dinner	Quickest Ever Spinach & Chickpea Curry	323	206

Total calories: **900**

Spare calories: 700 woman / 1,100 man

Why not try	Apple & Raspberry Cake	269	246

The Recipes

REGULAR DAY COMBO 8

		Cals/serving	Page
Breakfast	Avocado, Parmesan & Lemon Juice (on toast)	229	118
Lunch	Salmon & Prawn Chowder	299	194
Dinner	Harissa-spiced Pork Tenderloin with Roast Apples	336	208

Total calories: **864**

Spare calories: **736** woman / **1,136** man

Why not try	Poached Passion Fruit Pears	204	238

REGULAR DAY COMBO 9

		Cals/serving	Page
Breakfast	Boiled Egg, Avocado & Watercress (Stuff on Toast)	254	120
Lunch	Roast Asparagus with Grilled Halloumi, Orange & Almonds	349	211
Dinner	Lamb Curry Fake-away	452	224

Total calories: **1055**

Spare calories: **545** woman / **945** man

Why not try	Baked Stone Fruits with Spiced Yogurt	205	240

REGULAR DAY COMBO 10

		Cals/serving	Page
Breakfast	Sautéed Paprika Peppers, Goat's Cheese & Egg (Stuff on Toast)	286	120
Lunch	Hearty Veggie Soba Miso Soup	260	178
Dinner	Tandoori Whole Roast Chicken with Spicy Potatoes	683	230

Total calories: **1229**

Spare calories: **371** woman / **771** man

Why not try	Roasted Figs with Dark Chocolate Drizzle	212	242

The Four-Week Meal Plan

If you prefer all the work to be done for you, the easiest way to stick to the Midlife Method is with my Four-Week Meal Plan.

To recap:

- Week 1 – six Light Days/one Regular Day
- Week 2 – five Light Days/two Regular Days
- Week 3 – four Light Days/three Regular Days
- Week 4 – three Light Days/four Regular Days.

The meal plans have been designed to hit the calorie targets for Light and Regular Days as well as to be balanced across the food groups. Of course, if there are recipes you aren't keen on, simply swap them for something else with a similar calorie count.

For ease, I have assumed that the plans begin on a Monday. To get a head start on the week, some meal prep on a Sunday really pays off, so I've indicated at the start of each week which recipes can be made ahead, should you have the time/inclination to do so.

Like the meal combos, the weekly meal plans tell you how many calories you have spare per day. You can use these for sides, snacks – or, usually, in my case, a glass of wine. I would try to avoid snacking or drinking anything other than tea or coffee (with a splash of milk) and water on Light Days, as there really aren't many calories to play with. On Regular Days there is more wiggle room for those extras.

The only other thing to note is that you can do your Light and Regular Days in any order you wish. The number of Light Days reduces over the four weeks, and I have assumed that for most people it's better to have Regular Days at the weekend, but you can swap them around to suit your schedule.

MEAL PLAN FOR WEEK 1
– Six Light Days/One Regular Day

Meal prep

Here are the recipes for this week that can be made in advance:

- My Go-to Granola (p. 89)

- Rhubarb, Apple & Ginger Compote (p. 84)

- Pintopeño Dip (p. 124)

- Aubergine, Lentil, Red Pepper & Olive Stew (p. 202)

- Potato, Leek & Fennel Soup with Stilton (p. 150)

- Quickest Ever Spinach & Chickpea Curry (p. 206).

If you are starting on a Monday, it would be good to make the granola, compote and dip on Sunday so you are ready to go.

Meal plan

DAY 1 – LIGHT DAY			
		Cals/serving	Page
Breakfast	My Go-to Granola with Rhubarb, Apple & Ginger Compote, served with 2 tbsp Greek yogurt	225	89
Lunch	A wholemeal pitta stuffed with a serving of Pintopeño Dip and 100g mixed salad	209	124
Dinner	Tagliata & Watercress with a Mustard Orange Dressing	298	190

Total calories: **732**

Spare calories: **68**

DAY 2 – LIGHT DAY

		Cals/serving	Page
Breakfast	My Go-to Granola with Rhubarb, Apple & Ginger Compote, served with 2 tbsp Greek yogurt	225	89
Lunch	Shredded Brussels & Parmesan Salad	208	158
Dinner	Aubergine, Lentil, Red Pepper & Olive Stew	313	202

Total calories: **746**

Spare calories: **54**

DAY 3 – LIGHT DAY

		Cals/serving	Page
Breakfast	Stuff on Toast (choose any under 200 cals)	200	118
Lunch	Quick Lunch Assembly – Quick Chickpea Salad	210	197
Dinner	Fast Fish Pie	278	186

Total calories: **688**

Spare calories: **112**

DAY 4 – LIGHT DAY

		Cals/serving	Page
Breakfast	Quick Breakfast Assembly (choose any under 250 cals)	250	115
Lunch	Potato, Leek & Fennel Soup with Stilton, served with a slice of grainy bread	291	150
Dinner	Roast Cod with Basil Sauce & Cherry Tomatoes, served with a side of blanched asparagus	206	148

Total calories: **747**

Spare calories: **53**

The Recipes

DAY 5 – LIGHT DAY

		Cals/serving	Page
Breakfast	Brilliant Breakfast Muffins (one muffin)	193	97
Lunch	Potato, Leek & Fennel Soup with Stilton, served with two oatcakes	281	150
Dinner	Black Bean Fritters with Avocado Dip, served with a grated carrot side salad	326	188

Total calories: **800**

Spare calories: 0

DAY 6 – LIGHT DAY

		Cals/serving	Page
Breakfast	The Healthiest Pancakes in the World	160	87
Lunch	Beetroot, Carrot & Apple Slaw, served with 100g cooked chicken breast	287	134
Dinner	Quickest Ever Spinach & Chickpea Curry	323	206

Total calories: **770**

Spare calories: 30

DAY 7 – REGULAR DAY

		Cals/serving	Page
Breakfast	Simple Smoothie Bowl	284	109
Lunch	Warm Spinach Salad with Feta & Strawberries	277	184
Dinner	Sriracha Chicken Tray Bake with Charred Lemons, served with a green salad and a medium-sized baked potato	508	213

Total calories: **1069**

Spare calories: 531 woman / 931 man

MEAL PLAN FOR WEEK 2
– Five Light Days/Two Regular Days

Meal prep

Here are the recipes for this week that can be made in advance:

- Indian Black Bean & Spinach Soup (p. 168)

- Beans Provençale (p. 162).

You will also need the following made up in advance as they are used in other recipes:

- Spicy Seeds Topper (p. 122)

- Rich Tomato Sauce (p. 128) (make a double batch for use in Italian Aubergines and Easy Spinach & Ricotta Wholewheat Cannelloni).

Meal plan

DAY 1 – LIGHT DAY		
	Cals/serving	Page
Breakfast — Oaty Miracle Muffins (one muffin)	167	93
Lunch — Indian Black Bean & Spinach Soup, served with a slice of grainy bread	333	168
Dinner — Spinach & Parmesan Crustless Quiche, served with a sliced tomato salad	234	154

Total calories: **734**

Spare calories: **66**

The Recipes

DAY 5 – LIGHT DAY

		Cals/serving	Page
Breakfast	Baked Bacon & Eggs with Asparagus Dippers	194	99
Lunch	Beans Provençale	210	162
Dinner	Italian Aubergines, served with a slice of sourdough bread	358	176

Total calories: **762**

Spare calories: 38

DAY 6 – REGULAR DAY

		Cals/serving	Page
Breakfast	Spinachy Baked Eggs, served with a wholemeal pitta	387	105
Lunch	Tasty Tuna Toast Topper, served with a sliced hard-boiled egg	283	160
Dinner	Easy Spinach & Ricotta Wholewheat Cannelloni (four cannelloni), served with a rocket salad	425	220

Total calories: **1095**

Spare calories: 505 woman / 905 man

DAY 7 – REGULAR DAY

		Cals/serving	Page
Breakfast	Mexican Breakfast Bowl	312	111
Lunch	Crushed Potatoes with Peas, Smoked Salmon & Fried Egg	365	215
Dinner	King Prawn & Pea Baked Biryani	405	217

Total calories: **1082**

Spare calories: 518 woman / 918 man

MEAL PLAN FOR WEEK 3
– Four Light Days/Three Regular Days

Meal prep

Here are the recipes for this week that can be made in advance. It's best to make double batches of these so they can last two days or you can freeze any uneaten portions:

- Apple & Carrot Basic Bircher (must be made the night before) (p. 95)

- Broccerino Soup (p. 144)

- Best Black Bean Chilli (p. 166)

- Green Lentil, Tomato & Watercress Soup (p. 138)

- Simple Veggie Tagine (p. 164).

Meal plan

DAY 1 – LIGHT DAY		
	Cals/serving	Page
Breakfast Apple & Carrot Basic Bircher (make enough for two days)	182	95
Lunch Broccerino Soup (make enough for two days), served with a slice of wholegrain bread	273	144
Dinner Baked Sweet Potatoes with Tzatziki	299	192
Total calories: **754**		

Spare calories: 46

DAY 2 – LIGHT DAY

		Cals/serving	Page
Breakfast	Apple & Carrot Basic Bircher	182	95
Lunch	Broccerino Soup, served with two oatcakes	273	144
Dinner	Best Black Bean Chilli (make a double batch for two days), served with 100g (cooked weight) brown rice	340	166

Total calories: **795**

Spare calories: **5**

DAY 3 – REGULAR DAY

		Cals/serving	Page
Breakfast	Stuff on Toast (choose any, it's a Regular Day!)	300	118
Lunch	Rainbow Ribbon Salad with a Tahini Dressing, served with a pan-fried salmon fillet (100g)	445	170
Dinner	Best Black Bean Chilli, served with a medium (150g) baked potato and a couple of tbsp of grated Cheddar cheese	395	166

Total calories: **1140**

Spare calories: **460** woman / **860** man

DAY 4 – LIGHT DAY

		Cals/serving	Page
Breakfast	Quick Breakfast Assembly: Greek Yogurt, Blueberries, Lemon Curd and Chopped Walnuts	210	116
Lunch	Green Lentil, Tomato & Watercress Soup (make enough for two days)	164	138
Dinner	Quick Smoked Mackerel & Butter Bean Fishcakes (three fishcakes), served with green beans	328	130

Total calories: **702**

Spare calories: **98**

DAY 5 – LIGHT DAY

		Cals/serving	Page
Breakfast	Big Mushrooms	210	103
Lunch	Green Lentil, Tomato & Watercress Soup, served with two oatcakes	254	138
Dinner	Simple Veggie Tagine, served with 100g (cooked weight) wholegrain couscous or bulgur wheat	325	164

Total calories: **789**

Spare calories: 11

DAY 6 – REGULAR DAY

		Cals/serving	Page
Breakfast	Power-through Porridge (any variation)	350	107
Lunch	Paprika Roast Cauli & Sweet Potatoes with Feta	308	200
Dinner	Simple Chicken Chasseur, served with cabbage and crushed new potatoes	622	222

Total calories: **1280**

Spare calories: 320 woman / **720** man

DAY 7 – REGULAR DAY

		Cals/serving	Page
Breakfast	Stuff on Toast (choose any, it's a Regular Day!)	300	118
Lunch	Spinach, Mushroom, Onion & Feta Flatbreads	200	156
Dinner	Harissa-spiced Pork Tenderloin with Roast Apples, served with yogurt dressed green beans and hasselback potatoes	520	208

Total calories: **1020**

Spare calories: 580 woman / **980** man

MEAL PLAN FOR WEEK 4
– Three Light Days/Four Regular Days

Meal prep

Here are the recipes for this week that can be made in advance. Again, if you make double batches they can last two days or you can freeze them and eat another time:

- Carrot, Lemon & Ginger Soup (p. 146)

- 'They'll Never Know' Veggie Ragu (p. 132)

- Lamb Curry Fake-away (p. 224)

- Salmon & Prawn Chowder (p. 194).

Meal plan

DAY 1 – LIGHT DAY			
		Cals/serving	Page
Breakfast	Power-through Porridge with Banana, Coconut & Brown Sugar	321	107
Lunch	Carrot, Lemon & Ginger Soup (make enough for two days), served with one crispbread cracker	220	146
Dinner	'They'll Never Know' Veggie Ragu, served with 100g (cooked weight) of wholegrain spaghetti	223	132

Total calories: **764**

Spare calories: 36

DAY 2 – LIGHT DAY

		Cals/serving	Page
Breakfast	Stuff on Toast (choose any under 200 cals)	200	118
Lunch	Carrot, Lemon & Ginger Soup, served with one slice of grainy bread	286	146
Dinner	Vietnamese-Style Chicken Salad	246	174

Total calories: **732**

Spare calories: 68

DAY 3 – REGULAR DAY

		Cals/serving	Page
Breakfast	Brekkie in a Hurry	317	113
Lunch	Puy Lentil & Tomato Salad with Goat's Cheese and Green Chilli, served with a fried egg	390	204
Dinner	Salmon Tray Bake with Pak Choi & Noodles	520	228

Total calories: **1227**

Spare calories: 373 woman / 773 man

DAY 4 – LIGHT DAY

		Cals/serving	Page
Breakfast	Chorizo Omelette	208	101
Lunch	Pot Noodles	260	180
Dinner	Flaky Curried Fish with one Flatbread, served with wilted spinach	265	172

Total calories: **733**

Spare calories: 67

DAY 5 – REGULAR DAY

		Cals/serving	Page
Breakfast	Quick Breakfast Assemby: Oatcakes with Tomato, Avocado & Feta	268	116
Lunch	Hearty Veggie Soba Miso Soup (with double noodles)	360	178
Dinner	Lamb Curry Fake-away, served with a spoonful of Greek yogurt and 100g (cooked weight) brown rice	577	224

Total calories: **1205**

Spare calories: **395** woman / **795** man

DAY 6 – REGULAR DAY

		Cals/serving	Page
Breakfast	Stuff on Toast (choose any, it's a Regular Day!)	350	118
Lunch	Salmon & Prawn Chowder	299	194
Dinner	Tandoori Whole Roast Chicken with Spicy Potatoes, served with a dressed green side salad	718	230

Total calories: **1367**

Spare calories: **233** woman / **633** man

DAY 7 – REGULAR DAY

		Cals/serving	Page
Breakfast	Spinachy Baked Eggs, served with a wholemeal pitta	387	105
Lunch	Roast Asparagus with Grilled Halloumi, Orange & Almonds	349	211
Dinner	Smoked Mackerel Bowl with Avocado & Curried Lentils	494	226

Total calories: **1230**

Spare calories: **370** woman / **770** man

Maintenance

Progressing towards your target weight

The Midlife Method is not a 'diet' in the traditional sense that it has a beginning and an end. It's a programme of change, so even though you've finished the initial four-week programme, it's really just the beginning of a new way of eating.

Hopefully you've seen some progress: 5–7lb (2–3kg) in the first month would be a great result, a healthy and sustainable rate of weight loss. But remember, weight management is a continuous process. By applying the Midlife Method consistently – Light Days, Regular Days and the Midlife Method Healthy Habits – you will continue steadily towards your goal.

If you have followed the meal plans, stuck to the calorie allowances, kept active and worked on managing sleep, stress and alcohol and not lost any weight at all, it would be advisable to go and see your doctor or a dietitian, as there may be some underlying medical reason for this.

Even if you haven't lost as much weight as you had hoped – and weight loss will vary from person to person – you will most certainly be eating more healthily, which is an excellent result in itself, and your weight should continue to come down.

I suggest you weigh yourself once a week. If you are where you want to be, just do one or two Light Days that week for maintenance. If you still have more to lose, do three or four Light Days a week until you reach your target weight:

One or two Light Days per week for weight maintenance.

Three to four Light Days per week for weight loss.

HOW TO STAY ON TRACK

I hope that this book has inspired you to eat well, and you feel confident to continue with your healthier lifestyle. Here are some ways to stay on track and stay motivated:

- Seek out more nutrifoods that you enjoy – it makes supermarket shopping a lot more interesting.

- Experiment in the kitchen with new healthy, lower-calorie recipes, dig out old recipe books or search the internet.

- Spread the word: tell family and friends about the Midlife Method and get them involved too.

- Check out the Midlife Method website for more recipes and support (see the Resources section at the back of the book).

Even with the very best intentions it can be difficult to stay on track; our lives are busy and social occasions can throw a spanner in the works. Here are some scenarios that can nudge us off-course – and my suggestions for how to deal with them.

On flights

As the future of flying is currently 'up in the air' due to Covid-19, many airlines are rethinking their in-flight meal service. Indeed, most have dispensed with any kind of food provision on short-haul flights.

On longer flights some airlines are still offering meals, and it's worth remembering that you can usually pre-order special meals prior to departure, including healthier, low-calorie options.

You could also take your own healthy food and snacks: this is probably the best option.

Eating out

The first thing to say here is that eating out should be a pleasure, not a time to be agonising over what to eat, but if you eat out regularly – say, more than once a week – then it makes sense to think about your menu choices. Here are some tips:

- Pizza is OK (ideally the thin-crust variety), but share one with a friend and get a side salad to go with it.

- Avoid pasta with a creamy or cheesy sauce; go for a tomato-based sauce instead.

- Don't fill up on bread; have one piece then move the basket out of reach.

- If something is served with chips, ask if you can swap it for a salad. Perhaps order a portion of chips for the table to share.

- If you're ordering a main course salad, especially one with a thick, creamy dressing like a Caesar, ask for the dressing on the side so you can control the amount you put on.

- Drink plenty of water, as this will help keep your appetite under control.

- Eat slowly, enjoy your meal, and stop when you are full.

- Save desserts and cheese boards for special occasions.

On holiday

Holidays can definitely be tricky on the food front: a week or two where food and drink are the main event. You may well be on holiday with others and have little control over where you eat. My advice is, don't stress. Holidays are not the time to be thinking about weight loss, but equally you don't want to pile on the pounds. You will probably eat and drink more than usual but if you remember your Midlife Method 'Regular Day' Toolkit, you will still make good choices. To recap:

1. Eat with awareness.

2. Eat mainly nutrifoods.

3. Be calorie-aware.

4. Mind the macros.

5. Practise volume control.

These tips will also help:

- Try not to snack; save your food spend for meals. An ice cream or two won't matter, but don't overindulge just because you are on holiday.

- Stick to water or sparkling water. This will keep you hydrated and has no calories: juices, smoothies and mocktails all add up.

- If you drink, your alcohol intake will likely increase on holiday. See the Drink smart tips on p. 67.

- Limit desserts – fruit is your friend!

On special occasions

One of the best things about the Midlife Method is that you can enjoy special occasions, guilt-free. If it's Christmas, your birthday or an anniversary, have what you like and enjoy it – a few days a year won't make any difference to your weight. But your birthday doesn't last a week, and neither does Christmas. If you're going to have a big blowout on Christmas Day itself, don't also overeat on Christmas Eve and Boxing Day. A mince pie is fine; a whole box of Quality Street, not so much. Once the festivities are over you can easily get back on track with a few Light Days.

FOOD STRATEGIES FOR MANAGING FOOD CRAVINGS

Food strategies are simply ways of thinking about your own food issues and devising practical ways to deal with them in your daily life. We all have certain foods that we find hard to resist, or perhaps to stop eating once we start. Most traditional diets dictate that these foods are off-limits, but it's not realistic to deny yourself the foods you love to eat, and why should you? With the Midlife Method, nothing is off-limits but it helps if you identify your weaknesses and develop strategies for dealing with them so that you don't overeat.

Step 1. Identify your weaknesses. What do you love eating (or drinking) that isn't particularly good for you and makes you feel guilty for having it?

Step 2. For each item, assess when you usually eat it and why. For example, do you skip breakfast and then drop in to a coffee shop for a muffin on the way to work? Do you get home after the school run, or work, feeling ravenous and have a toast frenzy?

Step 3. Develop a strategy. For example, with the coffee shop scenario, have a good breakfast so you don't feel so hungry on the way to work – and walk on the other side of the road so you aren't tempted to pop in. If you are stuck in the habit of snacking after work, try having a glass of water and a piece of fruit a bit earlier, before the munchies kick in. A little bit of eating with awareness goes a long way.

The Midlife Method Cheat Sheet

You now have all the tools you need to lose weight and feel great. We've covered a lot of ground in this book and from time to time you might need a quick refresher of the key points, so here's a Midlife Method Cheat Sheet:

Light Days

800 calories

3–4 Light Days per week for weight loss

1–2 Light Days per week for weight maintenance

Avoid snacking and alcohol on Light Days. Drink plenty of water.

Regular Days

1,600 calories (woman)/2,000 calories (man) – or your own personal calorie allowance if different.

The Midlife Method 'Regular Day' Toolkit

1. **Eat with awareness:** Are you really hungry? What does your body need? Perhaps you're just thirsty? Eat consciously, not mindlessly.

2. **Eat mainly nutrifoods:** Eat mainly wholefoods or foods that are minimally processed, including plenty of whole grains, nuts, seeds, fruit, veg and good-quality lean protein.

3. **Be calorie-aware:** Think about the relative calorific values of the food (and drinks) you are consuming. You only have a set amount of food spend, so make it count.

4. **Mind the macros:** A balanced diet is key. Aim for roughly 30% fat, 25% protein and 45% carbs.

5. **Practise volume control:** How much are you eating? Don't overeat through habit; your body will adjust to being satisfied with less.

The Midlife Method Healthy Habits

Exercise: Aim for four or five 30-minute sessions a week, including a mix of high- and low-intensity activity, strength training and at least one longer session of aerobic exercise, such as an hour of tennis, cycling or running.

Sleep: Give yourself the best chance of a good night's sleep by improving your 'sleep hygiene' to include a regular bedtime routine and minimising screen use in the evening.

Stress: Learn how to recognise the signs of stress, and reset your expectations of yourself and of those around you. Exercise, meditation and eating well can help.

Alcohol: Stick to a maximum of 14 units a week and have no more than 6 units in one session. Have at least three drink-free days a week, ideally two consecutively.

What you have said about the Midlife Method

I've always been reasonably healthy in what I eat, but as I move through my forties, I have noticed that I can't have the portion sizes that I once had. It takes me much longer to shift weight and I get away with far less in terms of overindulging. I've also found that my palate has changed and I want to get as much taste and goodness as possible out of what I do eat. I love the Midlife Method recipes. They're easy to follow and use familiar ingredients, but often with a twist, which keeps things interesting. I can easily serve many of the meals to my family and friends and it doesn't feel like diet food. As a working mum of two boys I don't want to make lots of different meals. I also want to be able to feed my family well and not have them see healthy food as 'mum food'! Staying in shape/dropping weight is a definite incentive, but feeling energised, sleeping well and being able to do the exercise I enjoy is really important to me. I find that it's increasingly important to balance a range of factors but I want food to fit easily into my life without having to overthink it. The Midlife Method helps to guide me in all of this and keeps me on track. **Jo Irwin**

At 42, I found myself 3 stone heavier than I had been in my blissfully slim mid-thirties, with weight collecting on my middle as if it was a magnet. I was already waking up with hot sweats in the night and having irregular periods, and I felt that my forties had not started well! Faced with lockdown due to the Covid-19 pandemic, I texted a friend and told her 'This is my chance to get fit.' I still joined in the banana bread craze at first, because I find baking is very therapeutic, then I knuckled down and got started on the Couch to 5K running programme. I knew exercise alone wasn't enough, so when Sam gave me the opportunity to help with recipe testing for the Midlife Method I was over the moon. The first recipe I tried was Vietnamese-Style Chicken Salad and the vibrant colours, flavours and textures were just the kick-start I needed to get excited about healthy eating again. Each time I tried a recipe I thought 'This is never going to be enough' yet each time I found myself fully satiated and feeling great. This helped me see that, as a home cook who loves to feed people, my biggest problem is portion control. In a busy household the thought of 'going on a diet' just seems like one thing too many to think about, but the Midlife Method of taking a holistic approach to weight loss feels much more sensible, manageable and enjoyable! I think my forties are looking up after all! **Marie Rawlinson**

I'm one of those lucky people: I haven't had to worry about my weight since the age of 21, when my puppy fat left me (phew), then I lost more weight following each childbirth, exactly as my mother did! I do work very hard on my body: I exercise regularly and like to think I eat fairly healthily, but I like my food and drink. I have noticed that after the age of 45 (I'm now 48), maintaining my weight has been more difficult. If I slip with eating and exercise I notice I put weight on more easily, particularly on my tummy and thighs. I am conscious that I have to be more careful with what I eat – and the quantity! I like the fact that the Midlife Method recipes are tasty and filling and don't feel like diet food or abstinence (this suits me, since I have never had to think like this!). A holistic approach does appeal as my sleep patterns vary from great to very bad in reaction to stress, alcohol consumption and hormonal changes. **Emma McCallum**

Midlife weight gain just crept up on me. I had four children in my thirties and lost the weight after each one fairly easily. I got back to around 10 stone, which for me was comfortable, but in my mid-forties I suddenly realised that all my clothes were a bit tight and thought, 'How the **** did that happen?' For years I thought I'd eat a bit less and the weight will fall off, but it doesn't any more – so you definitely need to become more aware. I like that the Midlife Method recipes feel like 'normal' food: you can be vegan one day and a full-on carnivore the next and you don't feel that you are cutting out food groups. You talk about eating with awareness, and that's the key for me. I love the holistic approach the Midlife Method takes. Hurrah to you for coming up with something inspiring and something I feel I can work towards. Weight is the one thing in life you can control, but in a positive way, and I want to be good to myself and feel good, as I think we all do. **Katie Lynn**

Midlife hit me hard and very suddenly. It was a total shock. One minute I was fit, toned and I think (my husband may say something different!) a well-balanced human being, but all of a sudden my midriff expanded, my digestion was beyond sluggish, and on some days I found it a real effort to move. What amazed me about the Midlife Method recipes was that they didn't have huge numbers of ingredients, took little time to prepare, and they were full of flavour. When I think of eating healthily, I think of a huge shopping list, hours of prep and the flavour being blah. These were just what I needed: light, refreshing, and yet I felt I'd eaten enough. I really want to embrace the holistic side of self-care: I'm trying to integrate more exercise into my day because, as much as I hate it, I feel so much better afterwards. **Louise Lyle**

The Midlife Method recipes are fantastic because they are packed with flavour *and* low in calories. Before, it was either one or the other. Now I don't have to choose between eating what tastes good and eating more healthily. It's the best of both worlds! Cooking with ingredients I don't usually use has helped me understand that I don't have to eat grilled chicken salads all the time to lose weight. There are so many foods you can add to your repertoire, and Sam has made sure you'll enjoy all of them! **Peggy M.**

I am 52 years old and in the throes of the menopause. Until fairly recently I have managed to maintain my weight at a healthy level while not really thinking about it. But with the onset of menopause my weight has slowly started to creep up – my jeans are a bit tighter and I don't feel so confident getting into my bikini any more. I'm not sure if my appetite has changed, or whether I've gained weight because of a drop in my quality of sleep (due to occasional night sweats and those weird adrenaline surges that come with menopause), or whether my appetite for the odd glass (or two) of wine has increased. So for the first time in my life I'm watching my weight – not obsessively, but I am keeping an eye on what I put on my plate. The Midlife Method recipes are all healthy and packed with good things, but also really delicious and filling, I don't feel like I'm depriving myself of anything. And they are often quick to prepare, with relatively straightforward ingredients, so they're a doddle to make. **J.G.**

While I'm lucky that my weight has always been fairly stable, I now have to pay attention to each little gain before there's another little gain and I end up with the challenge of a big gain. The Midlife Method recipes have really shaken up the way I cook and menu plan. I love the straightforward methods: they always produce a tasty meal and contain useful serving tips to make the meal suitable for everyone – and the meals are requested again and again! I love the way the Midlife Method recognises how important exercise is in contributing to managing your weight. Looking at your overall well-being in this way has really had a positive knock-on effect on everything in my life, with the benefit of better sleep and lower stress levels. Feeling great makes each step so much easier to achieve and maintain. **Hilary D.**

Acknowledgements

I would like to thank the following superstars, who have acted variously as sounding boards, editors and contributors and have provided encouragement and positive vibes during the writing of *The Midlife Method*:

My husband Rich, for always being there with a reassuring word – and a glass of wine – when I need one.

My kids Rufus and Roxana for keeping it real – their favourite meal is still macaroni cheese.

My ever-supportive friend Mimi Spencer, who got me started on this mad midlife food journey in the first place and who has taught me so much about the business of writing.

My mum Stephanie (who tested many of the recipes) and my sisters Alex and Sophie (who didn't). I love you guys. Thanks for putting up with me banging on about healthy eating.

My fellow food writers in Singapore, Ghillie James and Alicia Walker, for your wise counsel and free editing services!

My nutritional consultant Sarah Schenker, whose professional scrutiny and insightful suggestions have been invaluable.

My excellent team of recipe testers, Jess Gale, Marie Rawlinson, Jo Irwin, Hilary Davis, Louise Lyle, Emma McCallum, Sara Strain, Zoe Prescott-Harris, Anjli Khurana, Vikki Ames, Katie Lynn and Peggy Mason – the recipes are all the better for your input.

And then there are the people who made this book happen: my agent Antony Topping at Greene & Heaton, who championed

The Midlife Method from the start and somehow sold the idea to the wonderful Lindsey Evans at Headline Home in the midst of a pandemic. To all those who have worked on the book – Kate Miles, Jane Hammett, Tara O'Sullivan, Lucie Sharpe, Jessica Farrugia, Tina Paul and Alice Moore – thank you for bringing my book to life.

Appendix

Calorie-counted sides and additions

When you have a few extra calories to play with, you might want to make some meal additions. Here are the calorie counts for some common side dishes, accompaniments and additions.

Vegetable sides	Calories	Serving size
Asparagus	20	per 100g
Broccoli	34	per 100g
Carrots	41	per 100g
Cauliflower	25	per 100g
Green beans	31	per 100g
Kale/greens	33	per 100g
Pak choi/bok choy	19	per 100g
Peas (frozen)	77	per 100g
Potatoes	77	per 100g
(one medium potato = 150g)		
Red cabbage	31	per 100g
Spinach	23	per 100g
Sweetcorn (frozen)	88	per 100g
Sweet potatoes	86	per 100g
White cabbage	25	per 100g

Fruit	*Calories*	*Serving size*
Apples	52	per 100g
Bananas	89	per 100g
Blueberries	57	per 100g
Cherries	63	per 100g
Figs	74	per 100g
Grapes	69	per 100g
Kiwi fruit	61	per 100g
Nectarines	44	per 100g
Oranges	49	per 100g
Peaches	39	per 100g
Pears	58	per 100g
Pineapple	50	per 100g
Plums	46	per 100g
Pomegranates	83	per 100g
Raspberries	52	per 100g
Strawberries	32	per 100g
Watermelon	30	per 100g

Salad sides	*Calories*	*Serving size*
Mixed leaf salad	25	per 100g
Sliced tomato salad	18	per 100g
Grated carrot	41	per 100g
Quick chickpea salad (p. 197)	210	per serving
Oil & vinegar dressing (to add to any of the above)	20	per teaspoon

Appendix

Grains/breads	Calories	Serving size
White rice	65	per 50g (cooked weight)
Brown rice	55	per 50g (cooked weight)
Quinoa	60	per 50g (cooked weight)
Bulgur wheat	42	per 50g (cooked weight)
Couscous	56	per 50g (cooked weight)
Wholegrain pasta	62	per 50g (cooked weight)
Homemade flatbreads (p. 156)	100	per flatbread
Wholegrain/sourdough bread	100	per slice
Wholemeal pitta bread	145	per pitta
Wholemeal wrap	119	per wrap
Oatcakes	45	per oatcake
Crispbread cracker	34	per cracker
My Go-to Granola (p. 89)	165	per 40g

Condiments/sauces	Calories	Serving size
Butter	34	per tsp
Olive oil	40	per tsp
Vinegar	1	per tsp
Greek yogurt (0% fat)	15	per heaped tbsp
Greek yogurt (5% fat)	24	per heaped tbsp
Mustard	4	per tsp
Horseradish sauce	20	per tsp
Soy sauce	3	per tsp
Sriracha	6	per tsp
Mayonnaise (regular)	31	per tsp
Lime or lemon juice	1.5	per tsp

Honey/maple/date syrup	17	per tsp
Spicy Seeds Topper (p. 122)	20	per tsp
Quick Berry Sauce (p. 86)	39	per 50g

Healthy meal additions	*Calories*	*Serving size*
An egg (cooked without fat/oil)	75	per large egg
Prawns	60	per 75g
Chicken breast (no skin)	165	per 100g
Pork medallions	135	per 100g
Salmon	208	per 100g
White fish	87	per 100g
Tuna	108	per 100g
Firm tofu	145	per 100g
Tempeh	193	per 100g

Drinks	*Calories*	*Serving size*
White wine	124	150ml
Red wine	127	150ml
Sparkling wine/champagne	89	120ml
Gin and regular tonic	124	25ml gin, 150ml tonic
Gin & slimline tonic	54	25ml gin 150ml, tonic
Lager	140	330ml, 4–5% ABV
Coffee/tea with milk	25	per cup
Latte/flat white (semi-skimmed milk)	126	tall/12oz/335ml
Cappuccino (semi-skimmed milk)	75	tall/12oz/335ml

Appendix

Resources

More from me

My blog: see www.midlifemethod.co.uk for more recipes and information on midlife health.

My Instagram account: see @midlifekitchen for daily motivation.

Weight management tools

The NHS healthy weight chart: https://www.nhs.uk/live-well/healthy-weight/height-weight-chart/

Personal calorie intake calculator: www.freedieting.com/calorie-calculator

For calorie count information and nutritional data

https://nutritiondata.self.com/

https://happyforks.com/analyzer

More low-calorie recipes

https://www.bbcgoodfood.com/recipes/collection/300-calorie-meal-recipes

Spencer, Mimi (2013), *The Fast Diet Recipe Book*. Short Books.

Spencer, Mimi (2014), *Fast Cook*. Short Books.

Bailey, Clare and Pattison, Justine (2019), *The Fast 800 Recipe Book*. Short Books.

Featherstone, Kay and Allinson, Kate (2019), *Pinch of Nom: 100 slimming, home-style recipes*. Bluebird.

Kerridge, Tom (2017), *Lose Weight for Good: Full-flavour cooking for a low-calorie diet*. Absolute Press.

Wicks, Joe (2016), *Lean in 15*. Bluebird.

Whinney, Heather (2017), *100 Weight Loss Bowls: Build your own calorie-controlled diet plan*. DK.

Free online workouts on YouTube

Sarah Gorman BlendFit

POPSUGAR Fitness

Lucy Wyndham-Read

Bad Yogi Yoga

Caroline Girvan

HASfit

Yoga with Adriene

Joe Wicks (The Body Coach TV)

Couch to 5K – free NHS running app: https://www.nhs.uk/live-well/exercise/get-running-with-couch-to-5k/

Meditation/calming/sleep apps

Insight Timer

Headspace

Ten Percent Happier

Hey Clarity

Calm

Lighthearts UK

Moshi

Alcohol-tracking app

www.drinkaware.co.uk/tools/track-and-calculate-units-app

Conversion Charts

Weight

25/30g	1oz	150g	5½oz	450g	1lb
40g	1½oz	200g	7oz	500g	1lb 2oz
50g	1¾oz	225g	8oz	600g	1lb 5oz
55g	2oz	250g	9oz	750g	1lb 10oz
70g	2½oz	300g	10½oz	900g	2lb
85g	3oz	350g	12oz	1kg	2lb 4oz
100g	3½oz	375g	13oz	2kg	4lb 8oz
115g	4oz	400g	14oz		

Volume: liquids

5ml	–	1 tsp
15ml	½fl oz	1 tbsp
30ml	1fl oz	2 tbsp
60ml	2fl oz	¼ cup
75ml	2½fl oz	⅓ cup
120ml	4fl oz	½ cup
150ml	5fl oz	⅔ cup
175ml	6fl oz	¾ cup
250ml	8fl oz	1 cup
350ml	12fl oz	1½ cups
500ml	18fl oz	2 cups
1 litre	1¾ pints	4 cups

Volume: dry ingredients – an approximate guide

Flour	125g	1 cup
Butter	225g	1 cup (2 sticks)
Breadcrumbs (dried)	125g	1 cup
Nuts	125g	1 cup
Seeds	160g	1 cup
Dried fruit	150g	1 cup
Dried pulses (large)	175g	1 cup
Grains & small pulses	200g	1 cup

Oven temperatures

°C	with fan	°F	gas mark
110°C	90°C	225°F	¼
120°C	100°C	250°F	½
140°C	120°C	275°F	1
150°C	130°C	300°F	2
160°C	140°C	325°F	3
180°C	160°C	350°F	4
190°C	170°C	375°F	5
200°C	180°C	400°F	6
220°C	200°C	425°F	7
230°C	210°C	450°F	8
240°C	220°C	475°F	9

Length

1cm	½ inch		8cm	3¼ inches
2.5cm	1 inch		10cm	4 inches
3cm	1¼ inches		20cm	8 inches
5cm	2 inches		25cm	10 inches

Notes

1 https://www.brainyquote.com/quotes/jane_fonda_467984.

2 'Obesity: Study of 2.8 million shows increased disease and death risks.' BBC News, 29 April 2019. https://www.bbc.com/news/health-48088391.

3 Kapoor, E., Collazo-Clavell, M.L. and Faubion, S.S. (2017), 'Weight gain in women at midlife: A concise review of the pathophysiology and strategies for management.' *Mayo Clin. Proc.* 92(10): 1552–1558. https://www.mayoclinicproceedings.org/article/S0025-6196(17)30602-X/pdf.

4 'Obesity increases dementia risk.' ScienceDaily, 2017. https://www.sciencedaily.com/releases/2017/11/171130133812.htm.

5 'Coronavirus: Does being overweight or obese affect how ill people get?' BBC News, 8 May 2020. www.bbc.com/news/health-52561757?ocid=wsnews.chat-apps.in-app-msg.whatsapp.trial.link1_.auin.

6 'Obesity Statistics.' House of Commons Library, 2019. https://commonslibrary.parliament.uk/research-briefings/sn03336/.

7 Arroll, M.A. and Atkinson, L. (2018), *The Shrinkology Solution*. Quadrille.

8 'Is longevity determined by genetics?' July 2020. https://ghr.nlm.nih.gov/primer/traits/longevity.

9 'Menopause does not cause weight gain, but increases belly fat, major review finds.' ScienceDaily, October 2012. https://www.sciencedaily.com/releases/2012/10/121016084938.htm.

10 Personal communication, 26 February 2020.

11 'Belly fat in men: why weight loss matters.' Mayo Clinic, 13 June 2019. www.mayoclinic.org/healthy-lifestyle/mens-health/in-depth/belly-fat/art-20045685.

12 '"My energy is back": How testosterone replacement therapy is changing men's lives.' *Guardian*, 9 September 2019. www.theguardian.com/lifeandstyle/2019/sep/09/my-energy-is-back-how-testosterone-replacement-therapy-is-changing-mens-lives.

13 Personal communication, 20 May 2020.

14 'Health benefits of indole-3-carbinol.' Thermography Medical Clinic, n.d. thermographymedicalclinic.com/health-benefits-of-indole-3-carbinol/.

15 Saljoughian, M. (2007), 'Focus on phytoestrogens.' *US Pharm.* 32(12): HS-27-HS-32. www.uspharmacist.com/article/focus-on-phytoestrogens.

16 Fetters, K.A. (2016), 'How much does your metabolism really slow over the years?' US News & World Report. https://health.usnews.com/wellness/articles/2016-09-23/how-much-does-your-metabolism-really-slow-over-the-years.

17 Hutfless, S., Maruthur, N.M., Wilson, R.F. et al. (2013), 'Strategies to prevent weight gain among adults.' Rockville (MD): Agency for Healthcare Research and Quality. Report No.: 13-EHC029-EF. pubmed.ncbi.nlm.nih.gov/23638485/.

18 Public Health England (2016), 'Government Dietary Recommendations.' https://assets.publishing.service.gov.uk/government/uploads/system/uploads/attachment_data/file/618167/government_dietary_recommendations.pdf.

19 Tedstone, A. (2018), 'Why we are working to reduce calorie intake.' https://publichealthmatters.blog.gov.uk/2018/03/06/why-we-are-working-to-reduce-calorie-intake/.

20 McCormick, R. and Vasilaki, A. (2018), 'Age-related changes in skeletal muscle: Changes to lifestyle as a therapy.' *Biogerontology*, 19(6): 519–536. www.ncbi.nlm.nih.gov/pmc/articles/PMC6223729/.

21 Harvard Men's Health Watch (2018), 'Preserve your muscle mass.' Harvard Health Publishing. www.health.harvard.edu/staying-healthy/preserve-your-muscle-mass.

22 Yuki, A., Otsuka, R., Kozakai, R. et al. (2013), 'Relationship between low free testosterone levels and loss of muscle mass.' *Scientific Reports*, 3: 1818. pubmed.ncbi.nlm.nih.gov/23660939/.

23 Bee, P. (2019), 'How to prevent middle-age weight gain: The science of staying slim.' Times2, The *Times*, 15 October. www.thetimes.co.uk/article/how-to-prevent-middle-age-weight-gain-the-science-of-staying-slim-3nf6bksw5.

24 Warner, J. (2005), 'Fitness level declines dramatically with age.' WebMD. www.webmd.com/fitness-exercise/news/20050725/fitness-level-declines-dramatically-with-age.

25 Arner, P., Bernard, S., Appelsved, L. et al. (2019), 'Adipose lipid turnover and long-term changes in body weight.' *Nature Medicine*, 25(9): 1385–1389. pubmed.ncbi.nlm.nih.gov/31501613/.

26 'Can you boost your metabolism?' MedlinePlus, US National Library of Medicine. medlineplus.gov/ency/patientinstructions/000893.htm.

27 Science News (2019), 'Why people gain weight as they get older.' ScienceDaily. https://www.sciencedaily.com/releases/2019/09/190909193211.htm.

28 Davis, C.D. (2016), 'The gut microbiome and its role in obesity.' *Nutrition Today*, 51(4): 167–174. www.ncbi.nlm.nih.gov/pmc/articles/PMC5082693/.

29 Mullin, Emily (2019), 'The bacteria in your gut may reveal your true age.' *Science*, 11 January. www.sciencemag.org/news/2019/01/bacteria-your-gut-may-reveal-your-true-age.

30 Cuesta-Zuluaga, J., Kelley, S.T., Chen, Y. et al. (2019), 'Age- and sex-dependent patterns of gut microbial diversity in human adults.' *mSystems*, 4(4): e00261–19. DOI:10.1128/mSystems.00261-19.

31 Merrell, W. (2018), 'The aging digestive system: Maintaining gut health as you age.' AgingCare. www.agingcare.com/articles/the-aging-digestive-system-maintaining-gut-health-as-you-age-211926.htm.

Notes

32 Rossi, M. (2019), 'Your 10-step gut makeover plan.' The Gut Health Doctor. www.theguthealthdoctor.com/all-articles/10-step-gut-makeover-plan-healthy-gut.

33 Deckersbach, T., Das, S.K., Urban, L.E. et al. (2014), 'Pilot randomized trial demonstrating reversal of obesity-related abnormalities in reward system responsivity to food cues with a behavioral intervention.' *Nutrition & Diabetes*, 4(9): e129. doi:10.1038/nutd.2014.26.

34 Teixeira, P.J., Silva, M.N., Matta, J. et al. (2012), 'Motivation, self-determination, and long-term weight control.' *International Journal of Behavioral Nutrition and Physical Activity*, 9: 22. www.ncbi.nlm.nih.gov/pmc/articles/PMC3312817/.

35 Personal communication, 15 October 2018.

36 US Department of Health and Human Services (n.d.), 'Appendix E-3.1.A4. Nutritional goals for each age/sex group used in assessing adequacy of USDA food patterns at various calorie levels.' health.gov/our-work/food-nutrition/2015-2020-dietary-guidelines/advisory-report/appendix-e-3/appendix-e-31a4.

37 Bouchez, C. (2013), '9 surprising facts about your stomach.' WebMD. www.webmd.com/women/features/stomach-problems.

38 Mok, A., Khaw, K-.T., Luben, R. et al (2019), 'Physical activity trajectories and mortality: population-based cohort study.' *British Medical Journal*, 365: l2323. https://www.bmj.com/content/365/bmj.l2323.

39 Howden, E.J., Sarma, S., Lawley, J.S. et al. (2018), 'Reversing the cardiac effects of sedentary aging in middle age: A randomized controlled trial.' *Circulation*, 137(15): 1549–1560. www.ahajournals.org/doi/full/10.1161/CIRCULATIONAHA.117.030617.

40 Age UK (2020), 'Osteoporosis.' www.ageuk.org.uk/information-advice/health-wellbeing/conditions-illnesses/osteoporosis/.

41 Hong, A.R. and Kim, S.W. (2018), 'Effects of resistance exercise on bone health.' *Endocrinol. Metab.* (Seoul), 33(4): 435–444. www.ncbi.nlm.nih.gov/pmc/articles/PMC6279907/.

42 Personal communication, 23 April 2019.

43 St-Onge, M.-P., Mikic, A. and Pietrolungo, C.E. (2016), 'Effects of diet on sleep quality.' *Advances in Nutrition*, 7(5): 938–949. www.ncbi.nlm.nih.gov/pmc/articles/PMC5015038/.

44 Patel, S.R., Malhotra, A., White, D.P. et al (2006), 'Association between reduced sleep and weight gain in women.' *American Journal of Epidemiology*, 164(10): 947–954. pubmed.ncbi.nlm.nih.gov/16914506/?dopt=Abstract.

45 Personal communication, 6 July 2020.

46 Chang, A.-M., Aeschbach, D., Duffy, J.F. and Czeisler, C.A. (2015), 'Evening use of light-emitting e-readers negatively affects sleep, circadian timing, and next-morning alertness.' *Proc. Natl Acad. Sci. USA*, 112(4): 1232–1237. pubmed.ncbi.nlm.nih.gov/25535358/.

47 Bisht, K., Sharma, K. and Trenblay, M.-E.(2018), 'Chronic stress as a risk factor

for Alzheimer's disease: Roles of microglia-mediated synaptic remodeling, inflammation, and oxidative stress.' *Neurobiol. Stress*, 9: 9–21. www.ncbi.nlm.nih.gov/pmc/articles/PMC6035903/.

48 'Signs of stress.' © Mind. This information is published in full at mind.org.uk. www.mind.org.uk/information-support/types-of-mental-health-problems/stress/signs-of-stress/.

49 'Stressed? Take a 20-minute "nature pill".' Original written by Tania Fitzgeorge-Balfour. ScienceDaily, 4 April 2019. www.sciencedaily.com/releases/2019/04/190404074915.htm.

50 Sunni, A.A. and Latif, R. (2014), 'Effects of chocolate intake on perceived stress: A controlled clinical study.' *International Journal of Health Sciences*, 8(4): 393–401. www.ncbi.nlm.nih.gov/pmc/articles/PMC4350893/.

51 'Alcohol: Balancing risks and benefits.' The Nutrition Source, Harvard/TH Chan School of Public Health. www.hsph.harvard.edu/nutritionsource/healthy-drinks/drinks-to-consume-in-moderation/alcohol-full-story/.

52 NHS (2018), 'Gallstones: Prevention.' NHS. www.nhs.uk/conditions/gallstones/prevention/.

53 The North American Menopause Society (n.d.), 'Drink to your health at menopause, or not?' www.menopause.org/for-women/menopauseflashes/exercise-and-diet/drink-to-your-health-at-menopause-or-not.

54 Parke, H., Michalska, M., Russell, A. et al. (2018), 'Understanding drinking among midlife men in the United Kingdom: A systematic review of qualitative studies.' *Addictive Behaviors Reports*, 8: 85–94. www.sciencedirect.com/science/article/pii/S235285321830083X.

55 John, E. (2019), 'Alcohol-specific deaths in the UK: registered in 2018.' Office for National Statistics. www.ons.gov.uk/peoplepopulationandcommunity/healthandsocialcare/causesofdeath/bulletins/alcoholrelateddeathsintheunitedkingdom/2018.

56 Sabia, S., Elbaz, A., Britton, A. et al. (2014), 'Alcohol consumption and cognitive decline in early old age.' *Neurology*, 82(4). n.neurology.org/content/82/4/332.short.

57 Drinkaware (2020), 'What is an alcohol unit?' www.drinkaware.co.uk/alcohol-facts/alcoholic-drinks-units/what-is-an-alcohol-unit/.

Recipe Index

Recipe Index

Recipe Index

General Index